BIRTHING BODIES
IN EARLY MODERN FRANCE

"This study, which explores a range of birthing bodies, female and male, and analyzes striking associations of texts, will be of interest to all those—not just sixteenth- and seventeenth-century scholars—who work on the complexities of sex boundaries and non-normative gender identities."

—Wendy Perkins, University of Birmingham, UK

The pregnant, birthing, and nurturing body is a recurring topos in early modern French literature. Such bodies, often metaphors for issues and anxieties obtaining to the gendered control of social and political institutions, acquired much of their descriptive power from contemporaneous medical and scientific discourse. In this study, Kirk Read brings together literary and medical texts that represent a range of views, from lyric poets, satirists and polemicists, to midwives and surgeons, all of whom explore the popular sixteenth- and early seventeenth-century narratives of birth in France.

Although the rhetoric of birthing was widely used, strategies and negotiations depended upon sex and gender; this study considers the male, female, and hermaphroditic experience, offering both an analysis of women's experiences to be sure, but also opening onto the perspectives of non-female birthers and their place in the social and political climate of early modern France. The writers explored include Rabelais, Madeleine and Catherine Des Roches, Louise Boursier, Pierre de Ronsard, Pierre Boaistuau and Jacques Duval. Read also explores the implications of the metaphorical use of reproduction, such as the presentation of literary work as offspring and the poet/mentor relationship as that of a suckling child.

Foregrounded in the study are the questions of what it means for women to embrace biological and literary reproduction and how male appropriation of the birthing body influences the mission of creating new literary traditions. Furthermore, by exploring the cases of indeterminate birthing entities and the social anxiety that informs them, Read complicates the binarisms at work in the vexed terrain of sexuality, sex, and gender in this period. Ultimately, Read considers how the narrative of birth produces historical conceptions of identity, authority, and gender.

Women and Gender in the Early Modern World

Series Editors:
Allyson Poska, The University of Mary Washington, USA
Abby Zanger

The study of women and gender offers some of the most vital and innovative challenges to current scholarship on the early modern period. For more than a decade now, "Women and Gender in the Early Modern World" has served as a forum for presenting fresh ideas and original approaches to the field. Interdisciplinary and multidisciplinary in scope, this Ashgate book series strives to reach beyond geographical limitations to explore the experiences of early modern women and the nature of gender in Europe, the Americas, Asia, and Africa. We welcome proposals for both single-author volumes and edited collections which expand and develop this continually evolving field of study.

Titles in the series

Women, Imagination and the Search for Truth in Early Modern France
Rebecca M. Wilkin

Imagining Women's Conventual Spaces in France, 1600–1800
The Cloister Disclosed
Barbara R. Woshinsky

The Ideas of Man and Woman in Renaissance France
Print, Rhetoric, and Law
Lyndan Warner

Intertextual Masculinity in French Renaissance Literature
Rabelais, Brantôme, and the *Cent nouvelles nouvelles*
David P. LaGuardia

Hermaphrodites in Renaissance Europe
Kathleen P. Long

Childbirth and the Display of Authority in Early Modern France
Lianne McTavish

Birthing Bodies in Early Modern France

Stories of Gender and Reproduction

KIRK D. READ
Bates College, USA

ASHGATE

Published by
Ashgate Publishing Limited
Wey Court East
Union Road
Farnham
Surrey, GU9 7PT
England

Ashgate Publishing Company
Suite 420
101 Cherry Street
Burlington
VT 05401-4405
USA

www.ashgate.com

British Library Cataloguing in Publication Data
Read, Kirk D.
Birthing bodies in early modern France : stories of gender and reproduction. -- (Women and gender in the early modern world)
1. French literature--16th century--History and criticism. 2. French literature--17th century--History and criticism. 3. Childbirth in literature. 4. Metaphor in literature.
I. Title II. Series
840.9'354'09031-dc22

Library of Congress Cataloging-in-Publication Data
Read, Kirk D.
Birthing bodies in early modern France : stories of gender and reproduction / Kirk D. Read.
p. cm. -- (Women and gender in the early modern world)
Includes bibliographical references and index.
ISBN 978-0-7546-6632-5 -- ISBN 978-1-4094-2499-4 (eBook) 1. French literature--16th century--History and criticism 2. Childbirth in literature. 3. French literature--17th century--History and criticism 4. Gender identity in literature. I. Title.
PQ239.R43 2011
840.9’354--dc22

2010043847

ISBN 978 0 7546 6632 5 (hbk)
ISBN 978 1 4094 2499 4 (ebk)

MIX
Paper from responsible sources
FSC® C018575
www.fsc.org

Printed and bound in Great Britain by the MPG Books Group, UK

A ma femme.
A mes filles.
For Camille, Hannah, and Alice

Contents

List of Figures

Acknowledgments

> [T]outes les bourgeoises prirent congé d'elle, avec toutes sortes de reverence et de courtoisie, et moy particulierement, qui sortis le dernier, et eus le bonheur de voir l'enfant dont est question et du quel on attent le baptesme. (*Les Caquets de l'accouchée*, 1622)
>
> [All the women took their leave of her, with all manner of bows and curtsies, and I in particular, who left last, and had the good fortune of seeing the newborn in question, whose baptism we await.]

This moment from the seventh day of the *Caquets de l'accouchée* provides an appropriate entrée into the thanks that are due to the many friends, family, and colleagues who have played a role in the gestation, birth, and nurturing of *Birthing Bodies*. The long-sequestered narrator, by turns witness to and embodiment of his cousin's own birthing body, implicates a community of support and the excitement and anticipation of reproduction that is dear to my heart. To the various midwives—readers, nurturers, listeners, editors, enthusiasts—my undying gratitude.

Erika Gaffney's unflagging support and prompt, professional response to each and every query makes her a midwife on a par with her celebrated early modern predecessor, Louise Boursier. Her skills were matched beautifully by the prompt professionalism of her editing colleagues across the pond, most notably David Shervington. The editorial acumen and generosity of Kerry O'Brien (aka "Lady Ashgate") bettered this project on every level, and her sense of humor saved my soul. Katherine Dauge-Roth and Rose Pruiksma were compassionate readers from the very beginning, and their confidence in my work remains invaluable; our intellectual ties were formed in the *ruelle* of the Colby, Bates, Bowdoin Early Modern Reading Group. Among these scholars I thank, in particular, Cristina Malcolmson and Charlotte Daniels, whose reactions were clarifying and transformative at important moments. Emily Kane's intellectual rigor and personal empathy remind me daily of the importance of abiding friendship in and out of the academy.

The models for collegial midwifery abound in my academic life. From my earliest, awe-struck apprenticeship in Renaissance literature with Nancy Vickers to the mentors to whom she guided me—François Rigolot and Natalie Davis—I have been most fortunate. At that same time, Anne Larsen provided a model of edition and analysis of women's texts to which I continue to aspire. This generation of generous, intellectual collegiality to which I can only pretend has been embodied for me most graciously in Kathleen Perry Long, whose capacious intellect, warm regard, and dedication to the field so impress me.

Given the rather long gestation of this work, I have had the occasion to see and evaluate many departmental and institutional arrangements with divergent levels of kindness and support. I am the luckiest of all: Dick Williamson was my first Bates mentor and a model of enthusiasm for scholarship in the context of a deeply committed teaching life. The longstanding and unflagging support of my cherished colleague, Mary Rice-DeFosse, the invaluable combination of playful and profound intelligence and sustaining friendship of Alexandre Dauge-Roth, and the unbridled positive regard of Laura Balladur have feathered my Bates nest most warmly. I treasure the collegial ruminations over couvade and maternal envy with friends Kathy Low and Lisa Maurizio that often preceded sumptuous meals with their loving families. To Jill Reich, Dean of Faculty, my great appreciation for her enthusiasm for my career, in and out of French; the Faculty Development grants through her office were of great assistance. I thank several librarian colleagues at Bates as well—Tom Hayward, Laura Juraska, and Chris Schiff—who performed great feats of research, retrieval, and translation on several important occasions. Will Ash provided patient and timely assistance with images. And finally, a warm thanks to Georgette Dumais, supportive on many levels, who saw and copied more versions of this manuscript than she might care to admit.

Having dedicated much of my scholarly life to feminist readings of women's work with many women mentors, it has been my great good fortune to be sustained by generous men as well, whose regard for my career and, more importantly, my heart made life so much more joyful: to Bruce and Dad, my supportive family of origin; to Stuart Malcolm, my brother of choice and friend of all time; to Bill Blaine-Wallace, brother of the soul; to Howard Rosenfield, confessor and beacon of hope, much love and thanks.

And last and most, my deepest gratitude to the women who most support and define my happiness in life: Edith Frey Read, whose birthing body gave me life and whose spirit, long delivered of its earthly cares, still guides my way; Hannah, my Women and Gender Studies daughter who reintroduced me to Judith Butler and others; Alice, student of bodies of all stripes (whose hushed exclamation at the pulpit of Saint-Etienne-du-Mont—"Dad, is that a pregnant man?!"—will stay with me forever); and always and forever Camille, the mother, wife, and soul mate who gave me this family and constant, patient, and abiding love.

***

A version of Chapter 2 appeared with the same title in *Esprit généreux, esprit pantagruélicque*: *Essays by His Students in Honor of François Rigolot*, ed. Reiner Leushuis and Zahi Zalloua (Geneva: Droz, 2008), pp. 141–58, and is reprinted with the kind permission of Droz. A version of Chapter 3 appeared with the same title in *Gender and Scientific Discourse in Early Modern Culture*, ed. Kathleen P. Long (Aldershot: Ashgate, 2010), pp. 259–77, and is reprinted with permission. A version of Chapter 4 was published as "Mother's Milk from Father's Breast:

Maternity without Women in Male French Lyric" in *High Anxiety: Masculinity in Crisis in Early Modern France*, ed. Kathleen P. Long (Kirksville, MO: Truman State University Press, 2002), pp. 71–92, and is reproduced here thanks to their kind permission as well.

In addition, the following institutions provided generous support for this book: the library of the College of Physicians of Philadelphia which, along with its Mütter Museum and its medical anomalies, provided numerous texts and distractions; the Houghton Library of Harvard University; Rauner Rare Books Library of Dartmouth College, whose friendly and helpful staff helped reunite me with my alma mater in ways they may not have known; the Bibliothèque Nationale de France; the British Library; and the New York Public Library, whose generous indulgence saved one very overwhelming day's visit from disaster.

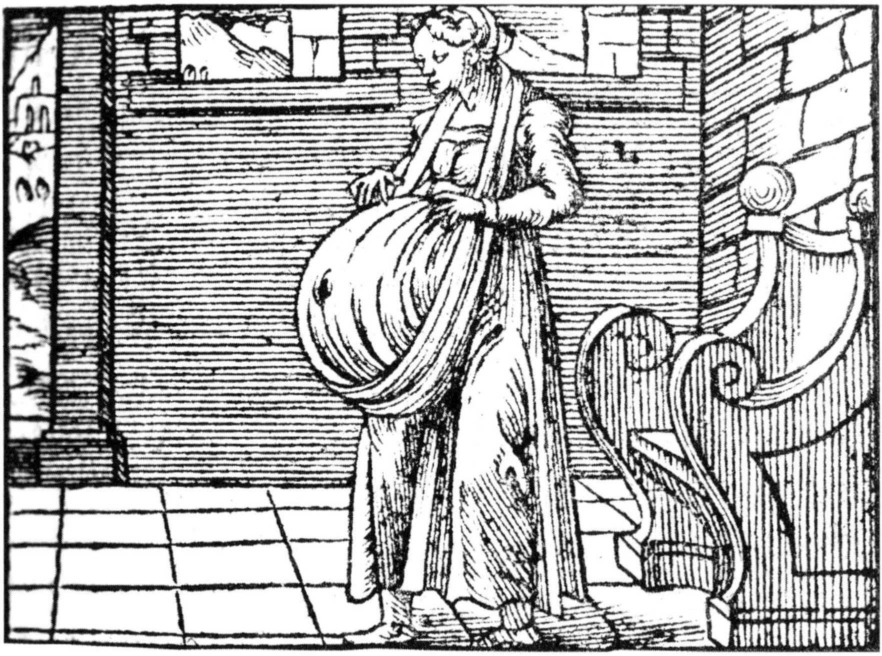

Figure I.1 Woman of multiple births, Pierre Boaistuau, *Histoires prodigieuses* (1597–8). Courtesy of Dartmouth College Library [GR 825. B63.1597. v. 2].

Introduction
Of Birthing Bodies in Early Modern France

Noz parens ont de loüables coustumes,
Pour nous tollir l'usage de raison,
De nous tenir closes dans la maison
Et nous donner le fuzeau pour la plume.

Bientost apres survient une misere
Qui naist en nous d'un desir mutuel,
Accompagné d'un soing continuel,
Qui suit tousjours l'entraille de la mere.

[Our parents have laudable customs
To deprive us of the use of our reason:
They lock us up at home
And hand us the spindle instead of the pen.

Then soon after comes a new misery
Born within us of mutual desire,
Accompanied by those continuous cares
That always burden the mother's womb.][1]

Madeleine des Roches, a learned widow living in mid-sixteenth-century Poitiers, published these stanzas as a lament over the ways in which women's literary lives were circumscribed by their birthing bodies and the patriarchal imperatives that governed them. The ode from which the lines are taken is her first poem in her first publication, following two dedicatory pieces ("Epistre aux Dames" and "Epistre à ma fille") and she is still in prefatory mode. Her voice in this work is at its strongest and most begrudging in terms of the travails of women and labors of various sorts. The ubiquitous and collective "nous" (and "noz") denote a clearly feminine constituency, communally condemned to the burdens of marriage and

[1] Madeleine des Roches in *From Mother and Daughter: Poems, Dialogues, and Letters of Les Dames des Roches/Madeleine and Catherine des Roches*, ed. and trans. Anne R. Larsen (Chicago, 2006), p. 53. All references to and translations of this work are taken from Larsen's *From Mother and Daughter*, with page numbers inserted parenthetically in the text unless otherwise noted. For Larsen's three excellent Droz editions of the des Roches works, see the bibliography.

family that draw women away from the life of writing. Further along in the ode she laments:

> Je voudroy bien m'arester sur le livre,
> Et au papier mes peines souspirer.
> Mais quelque soing m'en vient tousjours tirer.
>
> [I so long to spend time with my books
> And, sighing, cast my sorrows onto paper.
> But some distracting trouble always diverts me.] (55)

Distracted, diverted, Madeleine characterizes the mother's lot as onerous.[2] Torn between what is revealed later as great pride in her own daughter's accomplishments and bitterness over its cost, she condemns the society that has forced her into this life: "Il me suffit aux hommes faire voir/ Combien leurs loix nous font de violence" [It is enough if I can make men see/ How much their laws do violence to us] (55).

Madeleine's language in these stanzas betrays a woman who is acted *upon*, a woman to whom things happen, and who is not the agent of her own future. "Our parents" [Noz parens] from time immemorial, have customs that determine *us*, she says. Her syntax conveys this most eloquently in a repetitive, pronomial structure that underscores this dynamic of objectification. These laws deprive us [nous tollir], lock us up [nous tenir closes], and take from our hands our literary livelihood as they relegate us to domestic cares alone [nous donner le fuzeau pour la plume]. And from this scenario arises a life of misery, couched in a masterfully passive rhetoric that further defines the choiceless, voiceless young woman, now married, as the victim of her body and its social injunctions. Later, "comes a new misery," "born within us," and "accompanied by continuous cares" that issue from the mother's womb. The birthing body is unglamorously and unsentimentally rendered: for Madeleine, *mère* rhymes with *misère*.[3]

---

[2] I have chosen the not-uncontroversial option of naming the authors by their first names in order to distinguish them, and I have chosen not to overburden my prose by spelling out the entire name. One would seldom see Pierre de Ronsard or Joachim Du Bellay referred to as "Pierre" or "Joachim," for instance, but had they published with their progeny in such fashion, the conundrum would obtain to them as well, I can only presume. See Joan DeJean's treatment of this question in the introduction to *Tender Geographies: Women and the Origins of the Novel in France* (New York, 1991), pp. 41–4.

[3] I would refer the reader here to Figures I.1 and I.2 that I have chosen as illustrative of Madeleine des Roches's plight (and for the cover image for *Birthing Bodies*). This image of the spectacularly pregnant woman was ubiquitous in the period, reappearing in multiple versions and settings: posed here in the interior of the foyer of her home; lumbering about the countryside (a context similar to that of other medical and magical anomolies in, for example, Boaistuau's *Histoires prodigieuses*) and floating on the page, completely decontextualized in Ambroise Paré's complete works (see Figure I.2). The caption reads,

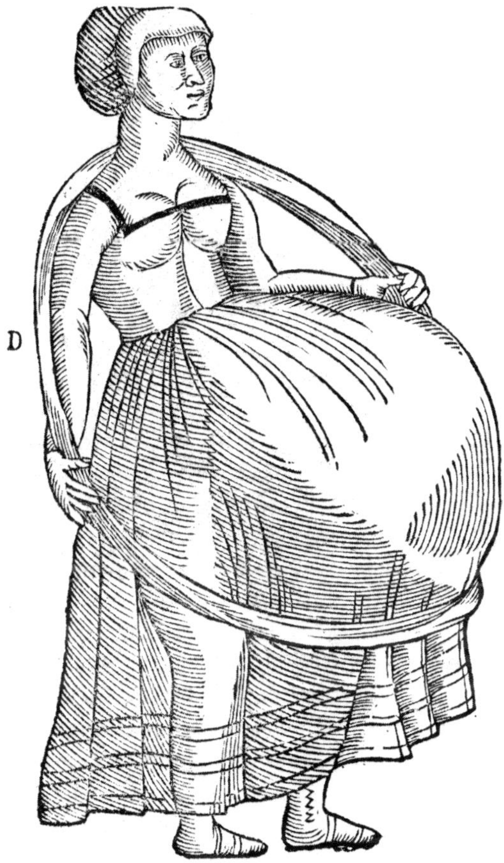

Figure I.2 Woman of multiple births, Ambroise Paré, *Les Oeuvres d'Ambroise Paré* (1633). Courtesy of Dartmouth College Library [R128.7 P2 1633].

All the more curious then, that the entirety of Madeleine's writing was published collaboratively with her very own daughter, Catherine. While Madeleine's first ode is a lament over the lot of women challenged by the misogynistic traditions that converge to impede their literary lives, her publishing history and her daughter's example are a stunning reversal of that sorry fortune. Witness the conclusion to Catherine's dedicatory epistle to her mother within this very same volume and how it responds to whatever she might see as the demands on her own body's birthing potential:

"Dorotheae multiplici sobole gravidae effigies" (Paré 1633). She appears by turns burdened, resigned, and even whimsically insouciant.

> [A]ussi n'ay-je point … laissé de mettre en oeuvre la laine, la soye, et l'or quand … vous me l'avez commandé. J'ay seulement pensé de vous monstrer comme j'employe le temps de ma plus grande oisiveté, et vous supplie humblement (ma mere) de recevoir ces petits escrits qui vous en rendront tesmoignage; si vous en trouvez quelques-uns qui soient assez bien nez, avoüez-les s'il vous plaist pour voz nepveux.
>
> [Thus I have not stopped working with wool, silk, and gold thread when you have asked me to. I have only thought of showing you how I employ my idle time, and humbly beseech you (my Mother) to receive this little collection of writing that bears witness to you; if you find some of them well enough conceived, please acknowledge them as your very own progeny.] (87)

Catherine shows herself to be every bit her mother's daughter: her prefatory epistle and the literary agenda she espouses over the course of her publishing career betray a woman responding to her mother's example in both life and literature. Here, Catherine recreates a feminized, literary universe in which her *mother*, who has just bemoaned her ancestors' ironically inflected "loüables coutumes," is the voice of authority to which she must appeal. Madeleine is betrayed as at least symbolically conventional, remanding her daughter, it appears, to engage in the most traditional of occupations for devoted daughters, that of spinning. Yet her obedience is in the service of a personally more satisfying calling: Catherine has been busy with the spindle, but the wool, silk, and gold that she has spun eloquently mark the progression from the mundane, domestic material of a woman's labor to the lustrous, literary pursuits that she is about to present.

Taken as a call and response of sorts, Madeleine des Roches's first ode and her daughter's epistle encapsulate several issues for literary women in language that is by turns touching, militant, and savvy. Her maternal, literary union with Catherine, with whom she publishes three volumes during her lifetime, is bittersweet indeed. Catherine is at once a precious companion and a reminder of Madeleine's wifely and maternal duties that do not always coexist felicitously: it is telling, for example, that the mother does not publish until such time as her daughter is old enough and sufficiently educated to include her work alongside her. Catherine's now famous sonnet "A ma quenouille" ["To my distaff"], which embroiders on the theme of the difficult prospect of holding both distaff and pen in the same hand, is part of this first collection and responds perfectly to her mother's heartfelt dilemma. The sonnet begins much in the same vein as her epistle, assuring the distaff—synecdoche of her patriarchal duty—that she is faithful to the proper work of her sex:

> Quenouille mon souci, je vous promets et jure
> De vous aimer tousjours, et jamais ne changer
> Vostre honneur domestic pour un bien estranger

[Distaff, my care, I promise you and swear
That I'll love you forever, and never exchange
Your domestic honor for a good which is strange] (111)

Here, Catherine is swearing allegiance to the domestic gods of duty whom her mother both represents and reviles, and then quickly makes a plea to this same audience for leniency and latitude:

Mais quenoille m'amie, il ne faut pas pourtant
Que pour vous estimer, et pour vous aimer tant
Je delaisse du tout cest' honneste coustume
D'escrire quelquefois …
Ayant dedans la main, le fuzeau, et la plume.

[But distaff, my love, it is not really necessary,
That in order to value you and love you so,
I abandon entirely that honorable custom
Of writing sometimes …
As I hold in my hand my spindle and my pen.] (111)

Catherine valorizes here another "coustume," a non-ironic invocation of a custom or tradition of women's literary pursuit that can marry her not to men, carnal desire, and the cares that issue from the womb, but rather to her mother, to the weaving of golden thread (poetry) and the immortality of *literary* progeny. "Distaff, my love," indeed. As we will discover later in more depth, Catherine eschewed marriage and the prospect of children of her own, despite a number of proposals. She embraced the literary life fully on her own terms and expressed her plan in a poetics entirely fitting for the daughter of a mother such as Madeleine, whose lament prepares her epistle quite logically. Catherine's writings are the ideal grandchildren for her literarily minded mother whose ode, in light of her daughter's witness, takes on the character of a manifesto. These children of the spirit are all the more "bien nez" for their proud, maternal lineage.[4] Not for Catherine these "continuous cares" that issue from the ingloriously rendered maternal womb.[5]

---

4 As Larsen points out, the "nepveux" is a clever play on words with Madeleine des Roches's birth name, Neveu, and also participates in a general usage of the term as referring to lineage, often in prefatory rhetoric, for male poets of the time, including Ronsard and Aubigné. Larsen, *Oeuvres*, p. 185, n. 11.

5 Madeleine's "entrailles" is a particularly pejorative term that Larsen translates fittingly through the use of "burden." Jean Nicot's *Thresor de la langue Françoyse* (1606) lists references to intestines and viscera only; the *Dictionnaire de l'Academie Française* (1694) provides the anatomical shades of "intestins" and "boyaux" along with the more general sense of "tous les visceres, toutes les parties enfermées dans le corps des hommes & des animaux." The figurative sense of parental bonding is presented as "Cette mere entendant

I begin this study of the early modern birthing body with Madeleine and Catherine des Roches because they set the stage compellingly for both the subject at hand and my own investigative trajectory through it. I will outline here and pay homage to my own literary ancestors, as it were, who opened both texts and contexts and helped bring into focus *Birthing Bodies*. Early work on the des Roches by Anne Larsen and later Tilde Sankovitch, along with an early study by Georges E. Diller two generations before them, is emblematic of the gynocritical mission of rescuing and making sense of women writers of the past, ignored precisely because of their gender.[6] My introduction to this mother–daughter pair grew out of this and other such pioneering work in feminist studies from the 1980s whose reassessment (or, in this case, rediscovery) of early modern women revealed these writers' astute negotiations of masculine poetics as they inscribed their voices in powerful, lasting, and imaginative ways. Madeleine and Catherine des Roches were exemplary in this way: their themes, their heroines, and their personal literary mother–daughter *ménage* contested the destiny of women relegated to biological reproduction and recentered their literary universe around women's prerogatives and potentials. Like their near contemporary, Louise Labé, the Des Roches's publications and lively, literary household bore witness to "assimilation with a difference"—to invoke the touchstone work on Renaissance women poets by Ann R. Jones—treading the line between familial and societal duty and the call to a learned life.[7] The last two decades of the twentieth century fueled a rich industry of editions, monographs, and anthologies aimed at fulfilling the dual missions of resuscitating lost or forgotten women's literary production and then putting this writing into theoretical constructs with particular attention to gender difference. Feminist literary and historical criticism of the early modern era established itself with rapid and prolific force. The critical voices from this era, many of which inform my work in *Birthing Bodies*, emerged in collections such as *Writing and Sexual Difference* (1982), *Beyond Their Sex: Learned Women of the European Past* (1984), *Rewriting the Renaissance* (1986), *Women in the Middle Ages and*

crier son fils se sentit toutes les entrailles émeuës," a characterization that alludes to "gut" instincts in a way more crude than other possibilities such as "ventre" or "matrice."

6 For my use of the term "gynocritical" I am beholden to the terminology coined by Elaine Showalter during this period in "Toward a Feminist Poetics" in Elaine Showalter (ed.), *The New Feminist Criticism: Essays on Women, Literature and Theory* (New York, 1985), p. 128. Much of Larsen's earliest work from this time has been incorporated subsequently into her excellent editions of the des Roches's *oeuvre* for Droz. Of note from this earlier period, "Catherine des Roches' 'Epistre A Sa Mere' (1579)," *Allegorica*, 7/2 (1984): pp. 58–64, and "Reading/Writing Gender in the Reniassance: The Case of Catherine des Roches (1542–1587)," *Symposium*, 41/4 (1987–88): pp. 292–307. See also Tilde Sankovitch, *French Women Writers and the Book: Myths of Access and Desire* (Syracuse, 1988), Chapter 2, and Georges E. Diller, *Les Dames des Roches: Etude sur la vie littéraire à Poitiers dans la deuxième moitié du XVIème siècle* (Paris, 1936).

7 Ann R. Jones, "Assimilation with a Difference: Renaissance Women Poets and Literary Influence," *Yale French Studies*, 62 (1981): pp. 135–53.

the Renaissance (1986), *Women in Reformation and Counter-Reformation Europe* (1989), and *Renaissance Women Writers* (1994). Important monographs such as those by Ann R. Jones (*The Currency of Eros*, 1990), Margaret King (*Women of the Renaissance*, 1991), Margaret Ezell (*Writing Women's Literary History*, 1993), and Merry E. Wiesner (*Women and Gender in Early Modern Europe*, 1993)—to name but a few from a large corpus—expanded this work while responding to a concomitant renewed attention to the edition, presentation, and translation of early modern women's writing by scholars on both sides of the Atlantic.[8]

If Madeleine and Catherine des Roches were influential for what their prolific literary output said of the opportunities and challenges for women negotiating a life in letters, their work also contained the specific reference, the person, to be exact, who was to redirect my focus on gender and writing in this period: Agnodice, the legendary first woman gynecologist, retold by Catherine in *Les Oeuvres* of 1579. As presented and contextualized in the third chapter of this book, Agnodice was a powerful touchstone for the connections between women's birthing bodies and literary production. In brief, Agnodice laments the plight of her Athenian sisters who find themselves fearful of the male doctors and compromise their health rather than reveal themselves so immodestly to their sight and touch. Agnodice cuts her hair, dons men's apparel, and goes off to study medicine, later returning to give succor to her suffering female compatriots. The myth is a marvelous metaphorical device for exploring the fate of women fearing male scrutiny and governance over their "corpus," be it anatomical or literary. The story of Agnodice allows us to investigate the confluence of the written and the writing body as informed by another strain of scholarship that has grown up alongside the feminist explorations of gender and literature, that of women as participants and patients in early modern medicine.

Historical work on midwives and doctors and the claiming of control over women's bodies in labor provides a fertile ground on which to appreciate the maneuvering of both women and men whose sources and discourses affect each other in ways that are by turns felicitous, nefarious, and most often a combination of both. Scholarly attention to the realm of early modern medicine and gender has been robust. A very partial list includes Valérie Worth-Stylianou's invaluable critical biography of obstetrical treatises from 1536 to 1627, *Les Traités d'Obstétrique en Langue Française au Seuil de la Modernité* (2007); several comprehensive works by Evelyne Berriot-Salvadore, whose more general *Les Femmes dans la Société Française de la Renaissance* (1990) narrows its scope to the medical in *Un Corps, un Destin* (1993); Jacques Gélis's much-cited *L'Arbre et le fruit* (1984), translated as *History of Childbirth* (1991), expansive in its reach and generalized

[8] Editions of women's works by Droz in Geneva, for example, and the tremendous service done to literary studies by the University of Chicago Press series, *The Other Voice in Early Modern Europe*, continue to present bilingual editions of women's work from this era. For full citations of the monographs and anthologies, as well as other works referred to in this introduction, see the bibliography.

in a desire to incorporate multiple sources from across three centuries; editions of the work of the midwife Louise Boursier by Françoise Olive (1992) and François Rouget and Colette Winn (2000), as well as the biographical work by Wendy Perkins, *Midwifery and Medicine in Early Modern France: Louise Bourgeois* (1996); Naomi J. Miller and Naomi Yaveh's *Maternal Measures* (2000), which includes a number of essays germane to the topic of birth and medical advice and control; Valeria Finucci and Kevin Brownlee's edited volume *Generation and Degeneration: Tropes of Reproduction in Literature and History* (2001), an indispensible collection for work on body and birth with a good deal of attention to the early modern era; the excellent study by Caroline Bicks, *Midwiving Subjects in Shakespeare's England* (2003), which does much of what *Birthing Bodies* hopes to accomplish in connecting early modern midwifery to literary concerns; and finally Susan Broomhall's *Women's Medical Work in Early Modern France* (2004) and Lianne McTavish's *Childbirth and the Display of Authority in Early Modern France* (2005), focusing on scientific and representational angles, respectively.

These studies betray an exciting, thorough, and abiding interest in recuperating and rereading a wealth of sources from across literary genres as they pertain to women's experience of medicine. What may surprise the reader of *Birthing Bodies* is the extent to which this book is concerned with men or non-females with regard to birthing, either through their physical bodies or metaphorically through literary appropriation. As my introductory example declares, it is women's experience that defined my stakes; over time, and given the revisions and recasting of questions of gender in the early modern era, the field of investigation has become only more expanded and instructive. And so to this albeit partial compendium of recent scholarship that privileges issues of early modern reproduction with regard to women's experience, I would add the exciting work of the last several years by scholars who extend discussions of sexed and gendered early modern writers into other areas, namely Kathleen P. Long's *Hermaphrodites in Renaissance Europe* (2006) along with her edited volume *High Anxiety: Masculinity in Crisis in Early Modern France* (2002), from which Chapter 4 of this book is largely taken; Todd Reeser's *Moderating Masculinity in Early Modern Culture* (2006); David LaGuardia's *Intertextual Masculinity in French Renaissance Literature* (2008); and Gary Ferguson's *Queer (Re)readings in the French Renaissance* (2008). Of obvious interest, if somewhat devoid of historical insight (because that is not his goal), is Roberto Zapperi's trans-historical compendium of men in childbirth, *The Pregnant Man* (1991). Sherry Velasco's study of the trope of the pregnant man in early modern Spain, *Male Delivery* (2006), compliments concerns that I explore in the French context, while opening up to a much broader contemporary application. Men as birthers, hermaphrodites, gender outliers, and women such as Catherine des Roches who refuse wedlock and the maternal imperative: such is the stuff of some of the most interesting terrain for conveying what is most salient and telling about how people of this era lived, negotiated, and navigated in their sex and gender through the domain of their bodies' actual and/or metaphorical birthing potential.

The example of the des Roches's mother–daughter virtual dialogue that I have only begun to address here, and to which I will return, is emblematic of the comparative approach that I will employ throughout these chapters. Mother and daughter nourish each other's writing, corresponding, responding, and expanding their literary universe in ways that may profoundly enhance our understanding of how writing and birthing bodies informed each other during this period. So too will I put their writings, and a host of other voices, in dialogue with a diversity of interlocutors—midwives, surgeons, and classical writers from their vast literary repertoire, among others—who might help to make sense of the power of their example. Finally, to their contemporaneous influences, I will add the voices of recent scholars whose investigations of birthing, sex, and gender constitute a now burgeoning field of inquiry to which this book hopes to add new ideas.

Evelyne Berriot-Salvadore defines her daunting mission in *Un Corps, un Destin* as the discovery of a gendered, scientific discourse in which women's lives were regulated and held in the balance:

> Plus attentif aux ouvrages spécialement consacrés à la médecine féminine, nous analyserons le développement de cette pathologie différenciée qui traduit une philosophie et induit une éthique. Mais, parce que le médecin est, de plus en plus souvent, un praticien qui observe la femme dans les vicissitudes de sa vie quotidienne, son témoignage mérite aussi d'être entendu: avec la gynécologie et l'obstétrique s'esquissent la destinée des jeunes filles, les souffrances de la femme mariée, le fardeau des mères.[9]
>
> [More attentive to works specifically devoted to women's medicine, we shall analyze the development of this differentiated pathology which conveys a certain philosophy and imposes a certain ethic. But, because the doctor is, more and more often, a practitioner who observes woman in the vicissitudes of her daily life, his witness deserves to be heard as well: within gynecology and obstetrics is outlined the destiny of young girls, the suffering of married women, and the burden of mothers.]

Berriot-Salvadore speaks directly to the *misère* inscribed in Madeleine's first ode and adds to the conversation the voices of the practitioners whose role in both treating and describing women's experience of birth was of crucial importance to their survival. The early modern male gynecologist outlines this destiny in ways that evince "suffering" and "burden," redolent of the conflicted issue of the "entrailles de la mère." Berriot-Salvadore's goal, as well as mine, is to interrogate these "differentiated pathologies," to visit the birthing body as a site whose discourses betray a complicated response to the primal potential of generation. Both doctors and midwives, whom Berriot-Salvadore does not ignore, present the generative

9 Evelyne Berriot-Salvadore, *Un Corps,un Destin: La femme dans la médicine de la Renaissance* (Paris, 1993), p. 2 (my translation).

body and their role in its oversight in telling ways, mining the past for inspiration and justification of their profession. Agnodice, for example, makes an appearance in Jacques Guillemeau's *De l'Heureux accouchement des femmes* (1609) as well as in Mauquest de la Motte's *Traité complet des accouchemens naturels* (1721), several generations later; Phanerote, the midwife mother of Socrates is implicated in Louise Boursier's proud lineage. The stories they tell about their *metier* and the women they service, when put into conversation with the more literary imaginings of the early modern era, offer a view to both men's and women's generative capacities that is at once sobering, liberating, and often unexpected. In this way, I depart from Berriot-Salvadore's dramatic, binary characterization—a body, a destiny—and strive to complicate or nuance what rings too often like a solitary, biological imperative. As I discover through the range of examples that I bring into dialogue, there are views to the birthing body that suggest a far from unitary birthing body and, indeed, a number of destinies.[10] A principal goal of *Birthing Bodies* is to reveal the ways in which the sharing and comparing of stories as told across gender, genre, and political agenda might nuance our understanding of the range of possible options for men and women of this era.

Methodologically, my approach is to investigate my sources, whatever their literary genre, as *stories*, tales of birthing, from conception to breastfeeding, with particular attention to the ways in which the corporeal realities of the birthing body find expression in writing according to an author's interests. Birthing stories, if one can be permitted some cross-cultural and trans-historical leeway, are most often dramatic, vividly rendered, crucial narratives that one tells to the world; as such, they also make for powerful metaphor. A number of mitigating factors may converge to heighten or inflect the drama of the birthing and lying-in: infant mortality; preferential gender treatment and aspirations; paternity (not to mention noble or royal lineage); virility, sterility, and fertility; the medicalization of the birthing process; and the anatomical (sometimes mortal) trauma that attends to early modern birth. Caroline Bicks underscores the power of birthing and storytelling well. In her essay "Midwiving Virility in Early Modern England," she delves into the vexed territory of women, gossip, and childbirth to reveal the drama that attends to female control over discourse, intercourse, and birthing bodies:

> Although there was a technical distinction between a midwife and a gossip—the latter being a friend or neighbor, but sometimes the child's deliverer as well—medical and literary texts often conflated these two figures and what they did together within the all-female birthroom. The gendered semantic shift of the term "gossip" and the conflation of gossips and midwives were part of a larger anxiety about the tales women scripted in this space … Whether or not they

[10] In a similar vein, Sara F. Matthews Grieco's *Ange ou Diablesse: La Représentation de la Femme au XVIe Siècle* (Paris, 1991) announces the binary *Zeitgeist* that, in my estimation, corrals texts and readings into reductive categories, all the more confusing and inadequate for explaining queer, hermaphroditic, or non-heteronormative examples.

> knew more than the husband or the state, birth attendants witnessed and testified to what few men could lay claim to having seen or known.[11]

Similar to Bicks's preoccupations, *Birthing Bodies* explores the convergence of the medical and the literary, as well as the anxiety over both women's bodies and women's discourse. I add to this the examples of men and hermaphrodites who inhabit this realm and recuperate women's reproductivity for their own purposes. These tales, scripted by and about a variety of subjects in childbed and put into dialogue—whether spun into alexandrines, carved into court documents and defenses, earnestly set forth in epistles as testimony or instruction, or parodied as "gossip" or in farcical gargantuan tales—reveal greater truths than any one isolated case. As Ann R. Jones investigated the "currency of Eros" across cultures, pairing women writers from throughout Europe, so do I ask here through some of the same processes of comparative reading: What is the currency of the birthing body in the early modern period? What are its vicissitudes? How is it scripted according to gender? What are its destinies? What is its meaning and value in the birthing of human life and of literature? What are its pathologies and agendas, its ethical and philosophical assumptions, in birthing and lying-in? What are its versions, its forms, its fictions and "facts," and what are the truths that are born from them?[12]

It becomes evident over the course of these chapters that the gendered universe is neither binary nor entirely predictable. It is my hope that the voices I engage with these narratives complicate rather than reify sex and gender boundaries. Lianne McTavish's astute observations of the gendered gaze with regard to birthing bodies of this period are particularly instructive:

> When scholars insist that women were increasingly exposed to an aggressive male gaze during the early modern period, they ignore the exhibition of male medical practitioners … This scholarship threatens to erase women from the picture by implying they were voiceless, passive objects lacking the power to resist. Obstetrical treatises written by both male and female authors depict, however, pregnant women who refuse to be seen. They also portray female midwives who intervene to mediate and even prevent male looking … These sources suggest that women's ability to look back, scrutinizing the bodies of male practitioners, should not be underestimated.[13]

---

11 Caroline Bicks, "Midwiving Virility in Early Modern England," in Naomi J. Miller and Naomi Yavneh (eds), *Maternal Measures: Figuring Caregiving in the Early Modern Period* (Aldershot, 2000), p. 50.

12 Ann Rosalind Jones, *The Currency of Eros: Women's Love Lyric in Europe, 1540–1620* (Bloomington, 1990).

13 Lianne McTavish, *Childbirth and the Display of Authority in Early Modern France* (Aldershot, 2005), p. 72.

Many of the early modern writers and stories we will investigate serve to nuance—looking back, talking back to—the sometimes flatfooted or overly invested readings of both feminist and misogynistic agendas. McTavish's work is salutary in this way, as are the revised readings of Galenic and Aristotelian anatomy by a number of scholars, most famously in Thomas Laqueur's much debated view of the one-sexed body and in the responses it has generated, notably by Katherine Park and Robert Nye, and more recently in Gary Ferguson's *Queer (Re)readings*.[14] Ferguson's work on homosexuality in the French Renaissance presents an erudite, generous, and apt approach when reading a variety of "queer" texts, many of which are taken up in *Birthing Bodies*, as the birthing subjects slip in and out of sexes and genders, though some evince more recognizable elements of homosexuality than others. Like Ferguson, I use examples that often privilege "textual moments that appear queer to the modern reader, that is, representations of various kinds that seem strange or sexually ambiguous, or that challenge contemporary heteronormative ideas and preconceptions." Ferguson continues (and I would join him in this enterprise), "Since such passages can often provoke in the modern reader a reaction of perplexity or embarrassment, giving them due attention, allowing their disturbing potential to unfold rather than seeking to explain it away, is already to foster a primary objective of queer theory" (Ferguson 51). Also common to my way into these challenging texts is the project of historical contextualization that considers the unusual instances of cross-gendering in the birthing process as unsettling, revealing, and liberating in terms of encrusted views of a binary sexual universe. As Ferguson proclaims, "The object of this second strategy of queer historical reading is clearly not to normalize the past, but rather to discover how it might be different from the present precisely in the ways it configured norms and marginalities differently" (51). Another touchstone in this regard that will have particular currency in my first chapter is the important essay on male menstruation during the early modern period by Gianna Pomata, her work serving as a radical revisioning of what medicine of the period had to say about health and norms in undeniably gynocentric terms. Reading early modern medicine with an eye to the body's surprising fluidity, and against the more popular grain of bodies destined solely to starkly predictable misery based on humors, proves liberating to both the scientific and literary potential of these authors and texts. As David LaGuardia cautions, "the most monolithic masculinity has always been structured in terms of its constant instability and undoing in the face of unquantifiable others that were beyond men's control."[15] Like LaGuardia, I value readings that dismantle received ideas about gendered bodies in early modern texts and mine them for the human

---

[14] Thomas Laqueur, *Making Sex: The Body and Gender from the Greeks to Freud* (Cambridge, MA, 1990); Katherine Park and Robert A. Nye, "Destiny is Anatomy," in *The New Republic*, 18 (February 1991): pp. 53–7; Gary Ferguson, *Queer (Re)readings in the French Renaissance* (Aldershot, 2008).

[15] David P. LaGuardia, *Intertextual Masculinity in French Renaissance Literature* (Aldershot, 2008), p. 13.

truths that reside precisely in that which is unstable and unquantifiable. Such an approach eschews too rigid a characterization of the gendered early modern world, and invites a more capacious view to the participation of all gendered beings in their multiple, negotiated, and improvised identities.

***

In Chapter 1, "Spying at the Lying-In," I investigate the hybrid literary phenomenon, *Les Caquets de l'accouchée*, published in eight installments over the year 1622. A complicated mix of parody, manifesto, particular history, and social commentary, *Les Caquets*, penned anonymously and by at least two separate authors, uses the birthing body as its framing device. The literary conceit is that of a melancholic gentleman seeking to recover from illness. He is advised to find for himself a recently delivered mother and to hide himself in the *ruelle* of the lying-in chamber. There, he is to record the gossip of the female visitors that will certainly regale him and return him to his "pristine santé." My close reading situates this text within the tradition of what might be called the "gossip genre," namely, medieval works such as the *Les Quinze joies de mariage* and the *Les Evangiles des quenouilles*, wherein men play a similarly beleaguered outlier to their wives' gynocentric *côterie* at and around the time of birth. In several of the *caquets*, the scribe fancies himself well steeped in the gynecological wisdom of his day, and I explore some of the contemporaneous references to which he may be alluding: his rather pedagogical aside on his own text as afterbirth [*arrière-faix*] prompts a reading of *Les Caquets* in this way and informs my thesis regarding the text as a nascent critique of salon culture, a view to the famous *ruelles* of the seventeenth century and their role in the production and critique of literary pursuits. If *Les Caquets de l'accouchée* has been rightly held up as participating in the age-old misogynistic tradition of the antifeminist side of the *querelle des femmes*, it warrants a reading as well that valorizes a certain view to women's productive and reproductive capacities, if at times unwittingly. I employ the work on the idea of male menstruation during the early modern period as a way of suggesting that texts such as these may well evince a more positive and inclusive view to women's creativity and procreativity than has been previously suggested—most notably by Domna Stanton in her work on *Les Caquets* as a "placental text."

Chapter 1 ends with a connection to one of the standard-bearers of women's reproductive health and a central figure in this book, the midwife Louise Boursier, whose livelihood was severely curtailed over the very question of afterbirth and a tragic lying-in. Chapter 2, "Staging the Competent Midwife," pairs a close reading of Rabelais's famous births of both Pantagruel and Gargantua with Boursier's dramatically rendered retellings of the births of Marie de Médicis, most specifically her first son, the future monarch Louis XIII. This chapter indulges most consciously perhaps, the phenomenon of birthing as an occasion for good storytelling: François Rabelais, as both chronicler and *savant* trained in medicine, and the midwife Boursier, who published a number of accounts and manuals—

most notably *Instruction à ma fille* to the daughter whom she hoped to see follow in her profession—tell entertaining accounts of dramatic births with literary savvy, great humor, and, most importantly, medical authority. While their accounts do not respond to each other literally, the literary and medical connections that are suggested deepen our sense of the valence of the birthing body at the royal level, be it the fantastical, gargantuan kingdoms of Rabelais, or the very real grandiosity of the French queen's elaborately staged and much scrutinized birthing chamber.

Chapter 3, "Touching and Telling," explores the professions of midwife and surgeon in greater depth through the literary imaginings of Catherine des Roches, quoted in the epigraph to this introduction. The mythological personage of Agnodice, the first woman gynecologist—who disguises herself as a man to be trained in medicine and return to the aid of her Athenian sisters—is the central character here. Using Louise Boursier again as the example of the flesh-and-blood equivalent of Agnodice, I compare versions of this story by Jacques Guillemeau—father to the royal surgeon who would ultimately judge and condemn Boursier—and Catherine des Roches. I subsequently compare them to the original tale as recorded by Hyginus (*Fabulae*, Gaius Julius Hyginus, c. 64 BCE–17 CE). Guillemeau's text comes from his popular medical manual, *De l'Heureux accouchement des femmes* (1609), and Catherine des Roches's "Agnodice" is found in her first publication, *Les Oeuvres* of 1579. The parallels between the ancient tale and the contemporaneous accounts are revealing with regard to the medicalization of the birthing process and the gendered control of women's health. Catherine des Roches rewrites this myth in a way that underscores the compromised lot of women described in the writings and example of Louise Boursier and prepared as well in des Roches's own literary discussions of gender, text, and (re)productivity that I have already partially explicated. My conclusion engages the turgid and anxious prose of an anonymous English translator of Guillemeau's text (*Child-birth or, The Happy Deliverie of Women* [1612]), whose trepidation before the blank page and the perceived shamefulness of women's birthing bodies invites comparisons with the early pioneering work by American feminists such as Susan Gubar and, especially, the radical manifesto of Mary Daly, aptly named *Gyn/Ecology*.

Chapter 4, "Assimilation with a Vengeance," turns to France's most historically venerated Renaissance literary elite, the Pléiade poets, to explore gendered, lyric permutations of the theme of nurturance, specifically breastfeeding as a metaphor for mentorship between Jean Dorat and his poetic disciples. If preceding chapters privilege the wisdom of surgeons and midwives and their writings on women's reproductive capacities, this section engages conceptualizations of the early modern body more generally. The much discussed work of Thomas Laqueur on the one-sexed body (to which I return in subsequent chapters) informs my reading of this curious trope on the postpartum birthing body that carries some of the resonances of the previous treatment of *Les Caquets de l'accouchée*, wherein men appropriate women's generative capacities (here explored through the metaphor of mother's milk as conveyance of language and art—*la langue maternelle*) as the woman all but disappears. The soaring, self-promoting mission of Ronsard and his contemporaries differs greatly from the parodic strains of the 1622 text, yet the investment in the procreative body remains consistent and perhaps more powerful when seen within a more capacious view of male and female bodies in flux. Just as Gianna Pomata's suggestion of the menstruating body as a healthy and purgative norm will help us reread the masculine appropriations in the imaginary afterbirth of *Les Caquets*, so does the view to early modern conceptions of anatomy complicate our reading of Ronsard and his contemporaries: as they subsume the female generative body into their poetic agenda, so do they valorize its potential for all writers, male and female, Catherine des Roches being, again, a prime example. She, too, eschews the messiness of the birthing body and recuperates the womb as a metaphor that allows a way out of, as Berriot-Salvadore suggests, *Un Corps, un Destin*.

The body in flux is at the center of Chapter 5, "Unstable Bodies," which turns to birthing as a potentially monstrous activity. This chapter furthers my exploration of the metaphorical usages of the birthing and nurturing body as played out in preceding chapters (namely "Spying at the Lying-In" and "Assimilation with a Vengeance") by taking up the confounding examples of what appeared to be men or male-identified subjects transgressing gender and sex assignments to actually give birth. The story that sets the scene here is Thomas Artus's *L'Isle des hermaphrodites* of 1605, a fantastical, dystopian text that serves as a thinly veiled critique of the corrupted court of Henri III. Here, hermaphodism fuels a critique of effemininity and sexual perversion as markers of political corruption. The author leads us onto a storm-tossed ship bound for a floating island of great instability, where the locals' comportment mirrors and extends this slippery, frightening, and inscrutable indeterminacy. I read this parodical text alongside contemporaneous works that take up medical anomalies, such as Pierre Boaistuau's *Histoires prodigieuses*—a hugely popular text from the previous century reprinted in multiple editions thereafter—as well as the more medically (and juridically) inspired *Des Hermaphrodits*, by the surgeon Jacques Duval. Hermaphrodite scholar Kathleen Long's important work on these texts greatly informs my investigation of this medical and literary phenomenon and prompts us to push further into a view to sexual ambiguity or transgression as perhaps the richest and most salient domain for expanding the discussion of birthing bodies as linked to social and political destiny. For what the stories of monstrous births of this period reveal about anxiety and indeterminacy, I also turn to the work of Judith Butler, whose discussion of gender illegibility, inscrutability, and regulation in *Undoing Gender* (2004) presents both the afterlife for these early modern conundrums and a theoretical construct for their reading more generally. This chapter delves not only into the ambient discourse on what appears to be masculinized birthing, but also into imagery, treating a number of visual representations in circulation during the early modern era that work in several directions, both reifying traditionally accepted biological norms and, at times, offering a more generous interpretation of the human body and its generative possibilities. The bisexual portrait of Francis I, for example, and Jusepe de Ribera's curious portrait of the bearded wife, Magdalena

Ventura, standing before her husband with her son at her breast complicate our assumptions about sex, gender, and generativity, again suggesting a way out of rigidly bifurcated gendered destinies.

The final chapter, "Strange Fellows in Bed," is a treatment of the phenomenon known as "couvade," wherein men suffer the throes of labor, delivery, and postpartum trauma alongside the women who actually birth their progeny. Originally conceived of as a conclusion to the first chapter on the postpartum scribe and his afterbirth in *Les Caquets de l'accouchée*, this study of explorers' accounts of indigenous societies serves as a conclusion to the entire book—a return to men spying, this time, at *men's* lying-in. A number of stories of couvade experiences surface in the narratives and reports of travelers, beginning with André Thevet in the latter half of the sixteenth century and reappearing in several seventeenth-century accounts thereafter. Here, the functions of the birthing body and its appropriation by men and/or male narrators are mapped onto a protocolonialist discourse wherein the transgression of one's sex and gender normativity is paired with (and amplified by) cultural otherness. As in the first chapter, I take my cues here again from a rich, fictional rendering of the couvade in medieval literature—Aucassin's encounter with the King of Torelore, lying in childbed as his postpartum wife storms off into battle in the "chantefable" *Aucassin et Nicolette*. Like Thevet and his early modern contemporaries, Aucassin finds himself in a land standing on its head. Confronted with a paradigm of the birthing body that challenges his gendered universe, he reacts with violence. Michael Wintroub's work, *The Savage Mirror* (2006), resituates this new world/other world discourse in the context of the staging of tribal tableaux for Henri II's entrée into Rouen in 1550, wherein the curious and confounding indigenous warriors, played by "true savages," inform a conception of the southern hemisphere as truly a world upside down. Many of the threads from the previous chapters are rewoven into this final chapter: just as the scribe from the *Les Caquets* spies at the lying-in, so does Thevet, flattened by illness, literally lie on the beach and report at one point on the strange couvade practices of the local tribes, their men also taking to (child)bed as their women return to labors of different sorts; in many ways, the arrival of French explorers on the shores of Brazil and on the islands in the Caribbean mirrors the fictional strains of *L'Isle des hermaphrodites* that might have more basis in lived experience than we might previously have expected; and these couvade accounts also make manifest, one final time, the connections between the birthing body, textual (re)production, and gender that have run through the entire book.

***

Earlier in this introduction I attempted to sketch out the critical voices that have helped shape my thinking about gender and literary production with increasing attention over the last several decades to medical and specifically gynecological discourse and wisdom. I take the opportunities traditionally afforded in prefatory rhetoric to make mention of a most formative influence in my own scholarly trajectory, the radical feminist Mary Daly. Her work *Gyn/Ecology*, written in 1978, was a fundamental act of repossession of women's bodies and health from the grip of what she saw as universally malevolent patriarchal control. Her self-consciously disruptive language cuts a wide swath across cultures and time periods in a way that is not particularly pertinent for my purposes here. Yet her impulse is. Her project is scheherazadian: retelling the stories of women, spinning their lives anew in a life-saving mission that is utterly and exclusively gynocentric:

> The title *Gyn/Ecology* is a way of wrenching back some wordpower. The fact that most gynecologists are males is in itself a colossal comment on "our" society. It is a symptom and example of male control over women and over language, and a clue to the extent of this control … Gynecologists fixate upon what they do not have, upon what they themselves cannot do. For this reason they epitomize and symbolize the practitioners of other patriarchal -ologies, and they provide important clues to the demonic patterns common to the labor of all of these.[16]

While the 30 years that have elapsed since the publication of this manifesto have seen undeniable progress in women's ability to claim self-determination with relation to health, Daly's prose is in many ways not outdated; it certainly harkens back to some of the men and women, givers and receivers of gynecological wisdom, that populate this book. Her view to de-pathologizing women's bodies and minds, to reclaiming a language that draws attention to inequity and attempts to move beyond it, and to negotiating, maneuvering, and seizing control still resonates with the texts and contexts of the early modern period and with my own project here. Daly's feminist agenda is one that constantly draws attention to heteronormative, sexist, and often racist assumptions about the "word of the Father." She witnesses and seeks to transform this inequity within the domain of women's bodies, bodies that call out for scripts and inscriptions, stories and contexts that privilege women's agency. We find these witnesses even in the early modern era—Louise Boursier and Catherine des Roches being our prime examples—and we find as well men whose participation in the realm of birthing bodies does not fall so neatly into the "demonic patterns" that Daly questions. There is surely evidence and example in *Birthing Bodies* to fuel this condemnation; there is also much that might nuance the pitched battle between matricides and patricides. My own livelihood depends on it.

Thirty years ago, I found myself in Mary Daly's wake as she stormed the Dartmouth College campus, then a bastion of the sorts of male demons she was calling out. I sat confused, a-mazed (her own term), angry (with her, with me, with my peers), and ultimately radicalized. Her virulent attack on the very institutions of patriarchy that both condemned and made room for her was transformative. Her playful yet violent recrafting of language so as to draw attention to itself, to

[16] Mary Daly, *Gyn/Ecology: The Metaethics of Radical Feminism* (Boston, 1978), pp. 9–10.

both its history of oppression and its liberational potential, transformed the way I studied language and culture. For much of the time she spent on campus she was sequestered, by her own demand and volition, in exclusively female community and conversation. She made a show of this exclusion and her public presentation announced that men would have no part in this gyn/ecological revolution. At her talk, men finally began raising their hands and she responded, "Well, I see there are no more questions." While I cannot pretend that there was not consternation, controversy, and more than a little self-righteousness, I ultimately turned toward, not away from, her truths. My doctoral work and much of my teaching and scholarship since have been devoted to communities of women of the early modern era, many of whom excluded male participation for reasons that, while they appear less radical, may well have addressed the very oppression Daly was attempting to mitigate 400 years later. *Birthing Bodies* introduces men into the gynocentric universe in a way that may not be uncontroversial, but it is my way in. What of men who attend to birth; who nurture in maternally defined ways; who appropriate generative capacities; who spy on birth; who envy, revile, embrace, and transform this fundamental moment? *Birthing Bodies* gives some historical perspective not only on the women whom Daly embraced during her storming of the Dartmouth campus, but also to the lives of those temporarily sidelined men who should, in my estimation, have an investment in this feminist agenda as well.

As this overview has suggested, there is a certain trajectory to the chapters in *Birthing Bodies* and a logic to the sequencing: we return in the conclusion (Postpartum), for example, to make observations on the first chapter with a similar text that I had reserved for this purpose. Nonetheless, the discrete chapters are meant to be able to stand on their own. To this end, there is some repetition in information (particularly on the Dames des Roches and Louise Boursier, who is somewhat of a starring presence in the book), but my hope is to have avoided redundancy. I have inserted references to pertinent chapters where possible to mitigate such problems.

***

In the epigraph that began this introduction, Madeleine des Roches laments the state of home-bound, duty-bound wives and mothers, "closes dans la maison" [locked up at home], followed in quick order by the "continuous cares" of her womb. Such might be an unglamorous depiction of her own lying-in, though her literary project would appear to be more about recuperating this regrettably burdensome turn of events with the prospects of (re)production of another sort. From her lying-in, then (to which we return in Chapter 3), to the anonymous male author of the early seventeenth century, whose surreptitious cooptation of the maternal space *par excellence* may deepen our understanding of the realm of birthing bodies in the early modern period.

Chapter 1
Spying at the Lying-In: *Les Caquets de l'accouchée* as Birthing Event

Les Caquets de l'accouchée, published anonymously as a series of eight pamphlets over the course of the year 1622, is the story of a man's labor at childbed. He has suffered through a terrible illness and the final plan for recovering his former health is curiously allied to a labor that is key to this book's concerns. "Nouvellement relevé d'une grande et pénible maladie" [Newly recovered from a great and painful illness], begins the narrator, "je fis assembler deux medecins de divers aages et diverses humeurs, qui, après m'avoir veu en bon estat, chacun d'eux dict son advis sur mon futur gouvernement et pour retourner en ma pristine santé" [I brought together two doctors of different ages and dispositions, who, each having seen me in a better state, gave their opinion regarding my future comportment so as to regain my original health].[1] His condition is suggestively "postpartum." He is recovering, but not back in full health, hoping to return to his pre-melancholic "pristine santé."[2]

---

1 *Les Caquets de l'accouchée: Recueil général suivi de l'Anti-Caquet, des Essais de Mathurine et de la Sentence par corps* (Paris, 1890), p. 7. This is the full collection of the *caquets*, which were published in eight installments (*caquets* or *journées*) in 1622 and then together as the *Recueil général des Caquets de l'Accouchée* in 1623. This edition (known as the *Recueil général*) includes the full complement of pamphlets (or *caquets*) published over several months in 1622, along with texts penned in response to these pamphlets, i.e., the *Anti-Caquet*, the *Essais de Mathurine* and *de la Sentence par corps*. When I refer to the *Recueil général*, it is to the 1890 text, which is an edition of the 1623 version. Translations are my own unless otherwise specified. All references are taken from this edition, with page numbers inserted parenthetically in the text. See also the edition by M. Edouard Fournier with introduction by M. Le Roux de Lincy (Paris, 1855); and an edition of the second *caquet* or *après-disnee*, in *La Seconde après-dînée du caquet de l'accouchée et autres facéties du temps de Louis XIII*, ed. Alain Mercier (Paris, 2003).

2 A brief note about the edition of the *caquets* to which this reading refers: As noted, the *caquets* were produced in installments throughout the year 1622. Opinion is divided over the uniformity of the authorship, but a certain fidelity to the conceit of the spying scribe and gossips gathered around the childbed is quite apparent. The author or authors betray an evolving sense of connection between the condition of scribe and the newly delivered cousin. It is this unfolding sense of connection and appropriation that I wish to exploit here. The editions that I have consulted are those mentioned in the previous note. A study of the metadiscourse of the editors who have attempted to streamline the authorial identity is not treated in depth in my reading; I take the arbitrariness of authorship as a given, while

The advice of the first doctor he consults is to repair to the country, smell the flowers, tour the gardens, enjoy a bit of claret, and then return to Paris on his mule, restored and in good spirits. The second doctor disparages this advice as too brief a cure and, in fact, possibly nefarious as it might prolong rather than assuage his *ennui*. He advises attending the theater—comedy, tragedy, or farce, all would suffice—perhaps from entertainments in vogue at the time by aristocratic children or, alternatively, travelling theater troupes from Italy (8–9). The first two bits of advice fail as the narrator is waylaid on the Pont Neuf (presumably on his way out to the country) by charlatans who attempt to swindle him out of his money—a chaotic scene of tricksters and farce of a sort that leaves him wondering if he has paid his consultants for naught.

And so on to the second doctor's final suggestion, presented as follows:

> Le second plaisir que vous prendrez (et qui est le meilleur), c'est de tascher à accoster quelqu'une de vos parentes ou amies, ou voisines, accouchées, pour vous permettre vous glisser à la ruelle du lict une apresdinée, pour entendre les nouvelles qui se racontent par la multitude des femmes qui la viennent voir, et en tenir bon registre; et par ainsi vous aurez non seulement dequoy contenter vostre esprit, mais aussi cela vous fera rajeunir et remettre en vostre pristine santé. (9)
>
> [The second pleasure that you might take (and this is the best), is to try to approach one of your relatives or friends, or neighbors who has recently given birth, who would allow you to slip into the alcove beside their bed some afternoon so as to hear the news that is told by the host of women who come visiting, and to write it down; in so doing you will have not only plenty to amuse your mind, but also the recapturing of some of your youthfulness and original health.]

Fate happily intervenes: this doctor has uttered the magical term "pristine santé" and the reader is alerted that this will be the true cure. As luck would have it, the narrator's cousin has been recently delivered of a child and he sets off to put the doctor's plan into action at her home in the rue Quinquempoix, which he cleverly (and fallaciously) rebaptizes "rue des Mauvaises-Paroles." Just two days after her delivery he arrives.

> Et, après avois congratulé l'accouchée, je la priay me donner ce contentement de me cacher à la ruelle du lict aux apresdinées, pour entendre le discours des femmes qui la venoient voir; ce qu'elle m'octroya facilement, à la charge de l'en dispenser si j'estois antiché de la toux, parce que pour rien elle ne voudroit cela estre descouvert. (11–12)

---

still recognizing the value and influence of previous installments and a forward trajectory through the lying-in period as the story unfolds.

> [And, after having congratulated the new mother, I asked her to do me the pleasure of hiding me in the alcove beside the bed in the after dinner hours so as to listen in on the stories of the women who came visiting; this she easily granted, on the condition that I would not importune her were I taken with a cough, for on no account did she wish for this plan to be discovered.]

Thus the narrator's plan is hatched with his cousin's consent. From the outset, then, the patient's cure associates the birthing body—here the postpartum body—with writing. While in the presence of his recovering cousin, he must not only listen in—a cure that would mirror the earlier, failed advice to take in a bit of theater—but also produce an account: he must "en tenir bon registre," write it down. Such a self-reflexive, writerly gesture validates his product, linking it not only to the gestational, generative potential of his cousin's "corps" become "corpus," but also to a tradition of literary works made from the stuff of nattering women and interloping males.

My trajectory through this reading of *Les Caquets de l'accouchée* proceeds in a way that attempts to emulate the very conceit that the text itself suggests, progressing through close investigation of the workings of *Les Caquets* through to my own "relèvement" of sorts that can bring the work to the light of scholars and theorists whose work may help make sense of this bizarre conceit. So, having presented the apparatus for this series of accounts of bedside confidences, I embed, as it were, this work in an established tradition of male literary "spies." I explicate the parallel conditions of the postpartum cousin and narrator as they evolve from their lying-in to their re-entry into society, their bodies consciously determined by theories of female humors circulating at the time. I then engage several theoretical approaches, literary and anatomical, that extend my close readings of the text in ways that may redefine this male appropriation of female generative capacities. For this, I turn to the early groundbreaking work of Domna Stanton on *Les Caquets*, as well as Gianna Pomata's important study of early modern conceptions of male menstruation and how a more gynocentric view to general human health might inform our postpartum narrator. Finally, I attend to the question of what exactly this man has birthed, engaging recent work by Faith Beasley and what it might suggest for *Les Caquets* as born out of a fledgling salon culture of the early seventeenth century.

A Tradition of Beleaguered Spies

At the close of the second day, the narrator is relieved to have a respite from the prattling as he is at the end of his resources. His reference here to the legend of the devil at the Mass of Saint Martin signals a tradition of gossiping women and scribbling male scribes that defines his project quite directly:

> [S]i elle y eut sejourné plus long-temps, il m'eut fallu faire comme le diable que vit un jour sainct Martin, qui, tenant registre derrière le pillier d'une eglise de tout ce que trois ou quatre femmes disoyent, et voulant allonger le papier qui luy manquoit avec les dents, de mal'heur il se frappa la teste contre le pillier. Moy, de peur que le mesme accident ne m'arrivast, j'ay mieux aymé remettre le tout à une autre fois. (86)
>
> [If she had gone on for much longer, I would have had to do as the devil did who was seen by Saint Martin one day; he was spied behind a pillar in church recording everything that three or four women were saying, and wanting to stretch out the dwindling margin of paper with his teeth, to his great misfortune, he cracked his head against the pillar. So I, fearing that the same accident would happen to me, much preferred putting it all off to another time.]

The scribe does not shy from comparing this behavior with sorcery—unsurprising, perhaps, as the milieu of midwifery and gossip is clearly and often associated with witches.[3] This reference to the scribe at Saint Martin's is a frequent intertext for men quarreling over women's loose tongues, and I will return to it at more length in the following chapter where Rabelais employs it to great effect. Perhaps most suggestive for our purposes here is the scribe's willingness to implicate himself as somehow "devilish," judging, but also colluding with the loose-tongued women in church. Such a conflation of the male and female condition and agenda is crucial to my apprehension of the text.[4] For the purposes of comparison here, however, two highly pertinent examples suggest themselves: *Les Quinze joies de mariage* [The Fifteen Joys of Marriage] (late fourteenth century) and *Les Evangiles des quenouilles* [The Distaff Gospels] (late fifteenth century); their preoccupations and associations with birthing and gender are particularly instructive.[5]

---

3 *The Malleus Maleficarum* (c. 1490) by Heinrich Kramer and James Sprenger is the often-cited ur-text for such associations. From Part I, chapter XI, succinctly put: "No one does more harm to the Catholic Faith than midwives. For when they do not kill children, then, as if for some other purpose, they take them out of the room and, raising them up in the air, offer them to devils." Ed. and trans. Montague Summers (New York, 1971), p. 66.

4 M. Le Roux de Lincy outlines the literary and historical context of lying-in narratives fairly extensively. See his introduction to the 1855 edition of the *caquets*, edited by M. Edouard Fournier.

5 As I investigate this trope of the cuckold, I must recognize David P. LaGuardia's work, *Intertextual Masculinity in French Renaissance Literature* (Aldershot, 2008), which, through a close investigation of three exemplary texts, treats the beleaguered male spouse as "an embodiment of a particular type of historically-contingent masculinity that is an essential element of late-medieval and Renaissance culture" (2). He continues, "In almost all cuckold stories, the supposed humor of the tale derives from the fact that 'the man of the house' has been 'unmanned' by his wife and her accomplices, who usually have as their goal the wife's sexual infidelity. The social being of this masculine personage was determined entirely by the diverse sets of laws governing marriage, which in turn were

Like the *Les Caquets*, *Les Quinze joies de mariage* springs from a tradition of misogynistic, satirical storytelling that opposes beleaguered men over multiple days as they navigate and record the inanities of gossiping women left to their own devices. In the third chapter of *Les Quinze joies* the narrator describes the now clearly ironic "joy" of attending to his wife in childbed: "après que le jeune mari et sa jeune femme ont goûté des plaisirs et des jouissances, lorsqu'elle tombe enceinte—et peut-être ne sera-ce pas de son époux, ce qui est un cas frequent" [after the young husband and wife have tasted of the pleasures and ecstasies and she becomes pregnant—perhaps not even by her husband, which is often the case].[6] The husband is run ragged, attending to each little whim of his increasingly feeble and demanding wife, and must play host to a panoply of visitors:

> Arrive le moment de l'accouchement: il faut qu'il fasse venir amis et amies, suivant le bon plaisir de Madame: alors il se fait beaucoup de soucis pour trouver ce qui manque aux amies, aux nourrices et aux sages-femmes venues là pour aider la femme tant qu'elle gardera le lit, et elles boiront du vin plus qu'une botte éculée n'absorberait d'eau. (37–8)
>
> [The moment of childbirth arrives: he must invite in friends, both men and women, according to his wife's bidding: he takes great pains to provide for all of the women's needs, for the nurses and midwives who have come to help out his wife for as long as she is in childbed, and they will drink in quantities large enough to fill an old boot.]

The author's conceit here is that the poor husband, likely cuckolded, is being duped at every moment: in English, the term "lying-in" might register on two levels. The continuous feasting and entertaining that the husband must provide (to his increasing financial ruin) is more about women's pleasure than pain. The wine flows freely and he is continually banished from women's company. As the drama unfolds, the husband and father-to-be is increasingly absent and maligned as he rushes about cooking up delicacies for his wife's cravings and his guests' overwhelming demands. At one point, the wife wails that her head is about to burst with pain, her suffering so overwhelming that she (insincerely) contemplates telling her women visitors to stay at bay.

> —Si, ma mie, dit-il, elles viendront et elles ne manqueront de rien.
> —Monsieur, dit-elle, laissez-moi tranquille et ne faites que ce que vous voudrez.

---

contingent upon the sexual usage that he made of his body in both civic and domestic space" (2). My preoccupation with the male figure as an appropriator of gynecological function and privilege takes me in a somewhat different direction, but I do find LaGuardia's work a valuable and beautifully theorized discussion of this comedic, gendered universe.

[6] *Les Quinze joies de mariage*, ed. and trans. Monique Santucci (Paris, 1986), p. 37.

> Alors arrive une des sages-femmes qui veillent sur la dame et elle dit à notre respectable benêt:
> "Monsieur, ne la contrariez pas en lui parlant, car c'est très dangereux pour une femme, faible, de petite corpulence et qui a la tête vide."
> Puis elle tire les rideaux qui entourent le lit.
> La dame ne veut donc pas se réconcilier avec le brave mari, parce qu'elle attend ses amies qui joueront bien la comédie. (44–5)
>
> [—But no, my dear, they shall come and they shall lack for nothing.
> —My lord, she says, just leave me alone and do as you wish.
> Then arrives one of the midwives who is looking after her lady who says to our dutiful half-wit:
> "Sir, do not contradict her when you speak, for it's dangerous for a woman so feeble, thin and lightheaded."
> She then pulls the curtains that surround the bed.
> The lady does not wish to reconcile with her brave husband, for she is waiting for her women friends who will play this comedy well.]

The wife and midwife are the producers in this drama whose comedic force obtains to all of the long-suffering husband's travails, certainly, but whose production depends on his exclusion: "Puis elle tire les rideaux qui entourent le lit" [Then she pulls the curtains that surround the bed]. One has the distinct impression that she and her consort of female visitors alone are allowed behind these curtains that are drawn against the gaze of the hapless husband. It is in just such a scene of domestic drama that the narrator of *Les Caquets* finds himself. His "register" of the women's gossip is, it could be said, the revenge of the husband of the *Les Quinze joies*: here, it is *he* who will hide behind the curtains in the *ruelle*. More connections with this text emerge in our reading of *Les Caquets*, but first a brief look at *Les Evangiles des quenouilles*, which inform this scene in similar ways.

Like *Les Caquets*, and similar to *Les Quinze joies*, *Les Evangiles des quenouilles* involves a group of women, a male narrator/scribe, and a sequenced narrative, here recorded over six nights via six female interlocutors. The text, a blend of antifeminist humor and late medieval folk wisdom, is parodic and ironic, with a broadly couched prefatory encomium to the esteemed female tradition into which these gospels will insert themselves—a flattery soon deflated once the stories are under way. The framing device alludes quite clearly to the *Les Quinze joies de mariage* (as well as the *Les Quinze joies de la vièrge*), the contemporaneous *Cent nouvelles nouvelles*, and is nourished by the tradition of Chaucer's *Canterbury Tales*, Boccaccio's *Decameron*, and prepares Marguerite de Navarre's *Heptaméron*. The narrator presents himself as an earnest defender of a glorious, though poorly documented female tradition of "doctoresses," citing Zoroaster's wife Hermafrodita as the initiator of these gospels and traditions. The tone quickly takes a turn as the "humble clerc" gets to his business. His project begins on one of the long evenings between Christmas and Candlemas:

> [J]e me transportay en l'ostel d'une assez ancienne damoiselle assez prez ma voisine, ou j'avoie acoustumé d'aler souvent deviser, car pluiseurs des voisines d'environ venoient illec filer et deviser de pluiseurs menus et joyeux propos dont je prenoie grant solas et plaisir. Mais pour ceste fois estoient empeschies de diverses raisons, et souvent de la grant haste qu'elles avoient de dire leurs propos, elles anticipoient l'une l'autre et parloient toutes ensemble. Moy, aucunement honteux de ceste ma soudaine avenue entr'elles, me voulz retraire arriere et pris congié d'elles en moy departant d'illec; mais soudainement je fus d'elles rappellez et de fait arretez par la robe par l'une d'elle, dont, moitié forcé, moitié requesté, je retournay et m'assiz entr'elles, et leur priay moult humblement qu'elles me pardonnaissent de ce que si franchement et si baudement me estoie embatus entre elles.

> [I went to the house of one of my neighbours, an old lady, where I often went to chat with several women of the neighbourhood who met there to spin and to exchange lively conversation, which I greatly enjoyed. That evening, the six women were present and very busy conversing, and because of their great eagerness to present their ideas, they interrupted one another and all talked at the same time. Somewhat embarrassed, because of my sudden intrusion among them, I wanted to withdraw and I bade them farewell and departed. But suddenly, I was called back and one of them pulled my robe so that half coerced, half cajoled, I returned and sat among them asking them very humbly to forgive me for having intruded among them with such liberty and boldness.][7]

This narrator distinguishes himself from *Les Caquets* by being implored by the women rather than hidden from them. In fact, however, much about the set-up heightens his otherness and perceived unwelcome in this milieu: while he has apparently listened in before on such conversations, when the women's banter becomes particularly heated, as in this instance, he feels entirely intrusive and out of place; his discourse is riven with alienation and a distinct sense of violation: he is "somewhat embarrasssed" [aucunement honteux] sensing a "sudden intrusion" [soudaine avenue]; he wishes to "withdraw" [voulz retraire]; "suddenly" [soudainement] he is called back, "half coerced, half cajoled" [moitié forcé, moitié requesté], and asks forgiveness for his "liberty and boldness" [si franchement et si baudement]. His satirical pose is that of being dominated by the women in this scene and the coerced/cajoled tension reads as a clear effeminizing of this man who feels himself in danger. The beleaguered husband of the *Les Quinze joies*, marginalized as he was as the women chattered on, is here redrawn as a victim of

---

[7] *The Distaff Gospels* [*Les Evangiles des quenouilles*], ed. and trans. Madeleine Jeay and Kathleen Garay (Toronto, 2006), pp. 72, 73. All references to the text and translations are from this edition.

more nefarious whims.[8] Having praised the glorious female tradition at the onset, he now appears less the humble, earnest scribe and more their slave. The set-up for the storytelling and introduction of the first of the "devisants" soon attaches this to the denigrated realm of gossip and midwifery.

The oldest of the six storytellers in *Les Evangiles*, Ysengrine du Glay, assembles her women and the narrator/scribe and begins by speaking in a cautionary vein about mistakes from the past: "les hommes du temps present ne cessent de escripre et faire libelles diffamatoires et livres contagieux poingnans l'onneur de nostre sexe" [men continually write slanderous satires and books harmful to our gender's honour] (74, 75). For a book that will do nothing but contribute to this slanderous satire, it is a shrewd move on the part of the author. Ysengrine then invokes the importance of this gynocentric literary event in a manner infused with references to lineage, descendancy, and conception. Of a shared, common humanity she suggests, "nous sommes fais tous d'un ouvrier, descendans l'un de l'autre" [we have been conceived by the same Creator]; she then genders this lineage with a promotion of female superiority: "sommes venues et descendues de plus hault et plus noble lieu qu'ilz ne sont, et faittes de matiere plus nette et plus clariffiee que eulx" [we originate and are created from a higher and nobler matter than they are] (74–6, 75–7). The work that the scribe will record will be their feminist legacy:

> a l'ayde de cestui nostre secretaire et ami, nous feissons un petit traittié des chappitres que volons tenir et mettre par ordre, lesquelz de pieça de noz grandes et anciennes meres ont esté trouvez, affin de les non mettre en oubliance, et qu'il puisse venir entre les mains de celles qui aincoires sont a avenir.
>
> [With the assistance of our secretary and friend, we should make a small treatise with the chapters that we want to develop and put in order—matters which have been discovered long ago by our grandmothers and our ancestors—so that they will not be forgotten and that this treatise can be passed on to the women to come after us.] (76, 77)

This is a heady and pointedly ironic passage, channeling the protofeminist, *querelle des femmes* mode of *Le Livre de la cité de dames*, by Christine de Pizan,

---

[8] James Turner's exploration of *Les Caquets* and similar texts underscores the sexual tension invoked as the male scribe penetrates the female sphere. Speaking of this example in the context of transvestment narratives, he states: "Male authors evidently felt compelled to don female disguise and penetrate, in imagination, that inaccessible world behind the façade of virtue, where women supposedly generate and transmit the truths of sex. Men wanted to regard themselves as the controlling source of all knowledge, the worldly authorities who inscribe their expertise on the blank and innocent female." Here in *Les Evangiles*, the parody relies on the monde à l'envers of women controlling, dominating, and determining. See James Grantham Turner, *Schooling Sex: Libertine Literature and Erotic Education in Italy, France, and England 1534–1685* (London, 2003), p. 53.

who summons within her treatise: "Vous qui êtes mortes, vous qui vivez encore et vous qui viendrez à l'avenir, réjouissez-vous!" [You (women) who have died, you who still live and you who have yet to be born, rejoice!][9] This from the author, we may recall, who announces her allegorical labor on the gynaceum as "bâtir et faire naître au monde une Cité nouvelle et éternelle" [to build and birth a new and eternal City] (47). The women of *Les Evangiles* assemble, led by Ysengrine:

> Dame Ysengrine du Glay y vint acompaignie de pluiseurs de sa cognoissance qui toutes apporterent leurs quenoilles, lin, fuiseaux, estandars, happles et toutes agoubilles servans a leur art. Et brief ce sembloit a veoir un droit marchié ou l'en ne vendoit que parolles et raisons, a divers propos de pou d'effect et de petite valeur.
>
> [Dame Ysengrine du Glay arrived, escorted by a number of her acquaintances who all brought their distaffs, flax, spindles, standards, reels and all the tools used for their art. In brief, it really looked like a market where nothing was sold but talk and discourse, conversations of little consequence and value.] (Jeay and Garay 78, 79)

This does not augur well for feminist evangelical wisdom, nor does the narrator's presentation of Ysengrine:

> Dame Ysengrine estoit eagie de .lxv. ans ou environ; belle femme avoit esté en son temps, mais elle estoit devenue fort ridee. Les yeulx avoit enfonssez et la bouche grande et large; cinq maris avoit eu sans les acointes de coste. Elle se mesloit en sa viellesse de recevoir les enffans nouvellement nez … Son mari estoit assez jone, duquel elle estoit fort jalouse et dont elle faisoit souvent grandes complaintes a ses voisines.
>
> [Dame Ysengrine was about sixty-five years old. She had been handsome in her time, but she had become very wrinkled; she had deep-sunken eyes and a big wide mouth. She had had five husbands not to mention her lovers. In her old age, she was busy delivering children … Her husband was quite young; she was extremely jealous and often complained about him to her neighbours.] (78, 79)

Ysengrine's midwifery seals the connection with the misogynistic tropes of gossip, birthing, women, and birth attendants that are part and parcel of *Les Caquets*. Her corporeal degradation mirrors her disreputability; she is a crone preying on multiple husbands and, it is presumed, women in childbed. This tradition of allying midwives with gossip and ill will is long and robust, as Caroline Bicks's excellent

---

[9] Christine de Pizan, *Le Livre de la cité des dames*, ed. and trans. Eric Hicks and Thérèse Moreau (Paris, 1986), p. 238.

work on this subject has shown. The force and longevity of this parodic strain is linked to the important issues obtaining to birthing and lying-in. As she states:

> Female birth attendants … compromised a man's position as patriarch when they moved into his household: they edged the husband out of his spouse's bed, sitting around it as the woman of the house entertained them both during and up to a month after the birth. Most importantly … the mother and her female attendants reminded the husband of his inferior powers when it came to telling stories about his spouse and her offspring. Their tales could initiate a story about a man's patriarchal identity (in its most literal sense) that might not match his own. Whether or not they knew more than the husband or the state, they witnessed and (in the case of midwives) testified to what few men could lay claim to having seen or known.[10]

The childbed is, therefore, a site of potentially life-altering witness, a tension that informs anxiety and frustration of the seemingly superfluous husband. Entrée into this female-controlled sphere, as in the unusual and privileged case of the narrators from *Les Evangiles* and *Les Caquets*, gives unique opportunity to regain control through appropriation of their private speech, characterized by Bicks and in these various examples as "telling stories." While the satirical strains of these fictitious imaginings plunge deep into humor, often of the most ribald sort, their power and poignancy is born of the deep personal and social stakes to which they are attached.

As evidenced in the discussion of these medieval literary precedents, the tradition of male narrators' appropriation of women's speech in which *Les Caquets* unfolds is, at best, ambiguous. But there is a richness and an opportunity for reinterpretation that may take our appreciation of the text to more nuanced gendered outcomes. Madeleine Jeay and Kathleen Garay's presentation of *The Distaff Gospels* is instructive in this way:

> The role of a man putting into writing what is presented as the oral tradition of women is a complex one, made even more so here by the presence of a double masculine influence: that of the author and his constructed alter ego, the scribe. Although he presents himself as their friend and ally, with a sense of superiority derived both from his gender and from his possession of literacy, the scribe nevertheless ironically distances himself from what he depicts as the ridiculous and trivial stories told by the women. (Jean and Garay 12)

They conclude later, "In the context of such recurrent and deeply embedded ambiguity, any attempt to focus only on the ironic antifeminism of *The Distaff Gospels* is to seriously over-essentialize this text" (18). I would agree and take this

---

[10] Caroline Bicks, *Midwiving Subjects in Shakespeare's England* (Aldershot, 2003), p. 25.

advice to heart in a treatment of such similarly ambiguous texts as *Les Caquets* that are their literary spawn. These authors can be seen as at once embracing the feminist strains of ancestors such as Christine de Pizan and deriding them in the ubiquitous discourse of gossip, babble, and sorcery so near at hand. Keeping this more generous and less bifurcated view to such troublesome tales may serve us better than more polemical interpretations. To uncover this fraught relationship between scribe and gossip, I turn now to these two postpartum entities as they converge in the shared terrain of the birthing body.

Parellel Postpartum Lives

As *Les Caquets de l'accouchée* opens, a large amount of time is spent, logically, preparing the setting in which the events will unfold. As the first visitors arrive at bedside, the narrator, attempting to emerge from his "grande et pénible maladie," settles into his perch behind a curtain in the alcove of the bedroom; his cousin's state mirrors this well: when addressed, it is her *mother* "assise proche le chevet du lict, à costé droict de sa fille" [seated next to the head of the bed at the right side of her daughter] who responds in her stead. "La fille accouchée rioit et n'osoit parler, luy ayant esté deffendu, à cause de la fièvre causée de la multitude de son laict" [The newly delivered daughter laughed and did not dare to speak, for she was forbidden to because of her fever brought on by the abundance of her milk] (*Caquets* 12). The incommodities of the first days of nursing known to any midwife, attendant, or observer of a woman in childbed are an authentic detail that plays nicely into the author's self-same dilemma: as the chattering continues on, his "production" becomes likewise troubled; the day ends with a reference to another of her physical needs that are mapped onto his dwindling resources; both are becoming a bit cranky with the lingering guests:

> [L]'accouchée, qui avoit envie de pisser, poussoit sa mère pour donner congé à tous; et moy, qui estois à la ruelle, qui manquois de papier et d'encre, me faschois de ne pouvoir tenir plus long registre de ce qui se passoit. (40)
>
> [The new mother, who needed to pee, nudged her mother to get all of them to leave; and I, in the alcove and running out of paper and ink, was getting annoyed at not being able to keep a more lengthy account of what was going on.]

Both the new mother and the scribe are in need of restoration, and as the second day begins, it appears that the cure is having its desired effect. The alliterative effect of "pisser," "poussait," "papier," and "ce qui se passoit" efficiently serves to bind their physical and literary incommodity.

The set-up for the second day portrays an even more philosophical narrator, waxing on about the restorative powers of social diversion:

> Comme ordinairement, aux maladies froides et humides, la melancholie y tient le premier rang, et que le seul remède de dissiper tous ses nuages, c'est de prendre une heure de passe-temps pour se rasserener les esprits debilitez … (41)
>
> [Ordinarily, with illnesses of cold and wet humors, melancholy is a primary symptom, and the only remedy for dissipating these clouds is to take an hour of diversion to calm one's failing spirits …]

The narrator reports the success of the first day of his cure, "qui m'avoit apporté quelque vigueur et quelque accroissement de santé" [which brought back some of my vigor and some renewal of health] (41–2). What is curious to observe in the narrator's gradual return to good health is his characterization of his melancholy as "froides et humides:" suffering in a state of cold and wet humors is also, according to Aristotelian-Galenic theory that held great currency in this period, a stagnation in the more natural state of women in general. Hot and dry was the natural, superior, and privileged domain of men; wet and moist was the lot of the changeable, unstable, and dark humors of women.[11] Indeed, the narrator makes explicit this state of affairs later as recorded in the "sixth day" (*La responce aux trois Caquets de l'Accouchée*), wherein the scribe speaks of getting into the baths to avoid the hot, dry sun:

> [L]es femmes, qui sont d'un temperament froid et humide, ne peuvent soustenir une chaleur si ardante que celle qui se fait quand le soleil entre au signe du Cancer, comme il a faict depuis quelques jours. (185)
>
> [Women, who are possessed of a cold and wet temperament, cannot endure so strong a heat as is produced when the sun enters the sign of Cancer, as has been the case for several days.]

As the scribe heals, banishing the specter of melancholy in his postpartum state, he moves progressively out of the biological sphere of women, even as he continues to claim its gestational power metaphorically. His connection to feminine humors is a specific medical reference that heightens the creative and procreative analogy.[12]

---

11 For a discussion of these humoral theories, see in particular Londa Schiebinger's chapter "Competing Cosmologies: Locating Sex and Gender in the Natural Order" in *The Mind Has No Sex?: Women in the Origins of Modern Science* (Cambridge, 1989), pp. 160–88; Thomas Laqueur's *Making Sex: Body and Gender from the Greeks to Freud* (Cambridge, MA, 1990); and Constance Jordan's *Renaissance Feminism: Literary Texts and Political Models* (Ithaca, 1990). See also Evelyne Berriot-Salvadore, *Un Corps, un Destin: La femme dans la medicine de la Renaissance* (Paris, 1993), pp. 23–31.

12 In a somewhat complicated progression of events occasioned by the hybrid nature of the "final" *Recueil*, the presenter of the sixth visitation of the accouchée is conceived of as a woman. To be clear, any progression or evolution I discern in *Les Caquets* is predicated

The male author is appropriating the condition of the newly delivered mother in ways that are increasingly flagrant, a gesture that Susan Stanford Friedman's early feminist work underscores as a decidedly political move as it relates to gender:

> The paradox of the childbirth metaphor is that its contextual resonance is fundamentally at odds with the very comparison it makes. While the metaphor draws together mind and body, word and womb, it also evokes the sexual division of labor upon which Western patriarchy is founded. The vehicle of the metaphor (procreation) acts in opposition to the tenor it serves (creation) because it inevitably reminds the reader of the historical realities that contradict the comparison being made. Facing constant challenges to their creativity, women writers often find their dilemma expressed in terms of the opposition between books and babies.[13]

Shades of Madeleine and Catherine des Roches. The narrator here can be seen (and indeed Friedman would see him) as intruding into the female space in ever more intimate ways—penetrating the lying-in chamber to report women's speech surreptitiously; taking on postpartum melancholy and ill humors; suffering the incommodities of lingering well-wishers more interested in their own prattle than his/her condition.

The third day begins with an account of the narrator's conversation with a doctor who has dietary advice for the newly delivered mother. The exchange betrays specific gynecological awareness:

> Depuis hier j'ay appris d'un certain medecin de mes amis que les potages blancs estoient grandement profitables aux accouchées … d'autant qu'elles ont besoin de restringens propres pour arrester le grand flux qui arrive aux femmes lors de leur accouchement, outre qu'il est besoin de les resserrer … Je fis mon profit de ce que me dit le medecin, pour le dire le lendemain à ma cousine. (87)
>
> [Since yesterday, I've learned from a certain doctor of some friends that white soups were highly salutary for newly delivered women … in as much as they need proper restringents in order to stop the large flow that women experience at the time of childbirth which they need to staunch … I took note of what the doctor told me and told it the next day to my cousin.]

The slippage between his own doctor who is prescribing the "listening cure," as it were, and this doctor of friends whom he apparently has engaged in some depth about women in childbed, is telling. He has clearly taken it upon himself to learn to

---

upon the final, redacted version of the ensemble, whose editing for uniformity is well outlined in the nineteenth-century editions.

13 Susan Stanford Friedman, "Creativity and the Childbirth Metaphor: Gender Difference in Literary Discourse," *Feminist Studies*, 13/1 (1987): pp. 49–82.

care for his cousin in very careful and pragmatic ways, contemplating postpartum flow, restringents, and diet. His care for her and for himself seem strictly aligned. After having arrived at his cousin's house and chatted a bit about their consternation with some of the preceding day's gossip, he sets to work: "Après luy avoir dict ce que j'avois apris de ce medecin, je me plaçay dans le cabinet qui est au chevet de son lict, et me mis là en estat d'escrire" [After having told her what I had learned from the doctor, I put myself in the closet at the head of the bed and got poised to write] (88). On the second day, the cousin has replaced the curtained-off alcove with "une petite estude, où l'on peut entrer par une petite porte" [a small study entered by a little door] (43). The "estude," now become "cabinet," prefigures the "cabinet de medecin," perhaps, as the narrator evinces here a more medically learned tone with regard to the recovery of his cousin which so mirrors his own. The newly recharacterized hiding place also clearly resonates with the scribe's reference to the marvels of the "cabinet de medecines" in the seventh *caquets* to which we will return in due course.

"Arrière toute melancolie!" [Banished all melancholy!] (117) begins the fourth day as both the narrator and the cousin fall into lengthy, intimate conversation: "ma cousine me receut à bras ouverts" [my cousin received me with open arms] (118). Their attenuated introductory conversation signals a growing health for both, a change remarked upon by one of the first arrivals: "Sans mentir, je te trouve plus belle que jamais. Asseurement, les enfans t'embellissent: je te conseille d'en recommencer un bien tost" [It's no lie, I find you more beautiful than ever. To be sure, babies are adding to your beauty: I would advise you to start again soon] (120). Soon after the gossiping visitors leave that day, the scribe bounds from his hiding place: "Je sortis incontinent après et me rangeay auprès de l'accouchée, pour luy monstrer mon ample memoire; je vous laisse à penser si ce fut sans rire" [I leapt out straightaway and took my place beside the new mother in order to show her my ample memoir; I leave it to your imagination as to whether or not we could contain our laughter] (145). The postpartum mother regains her health after having carried, "grown," and delivered her child; the visitations and banter, despite her occasional protestations, appear to be part of this recovery. The post-malady scribe appears to be delivering himself of his *own* work—an ample memoir—as a way of working through his melancholy. It is as though he himself is responding to the compliments and invitations of the admiring guests who lavish praise upon the cousin's increasingly healthful countenance, predicated, as they suggest, upon her productiveness. "Indeed!" the scribe appears to say, "Look at what we've produced!" The fact that the *caquets* are generated in successive installments is not inconsequential. The cousin has produced "cinq petites canailles" [five little rascals] (120) and, as the conspiring cousins head into the fifth day of gossip, their collaborative enterprise has generated a prodigious tome. Their (pro)creative scheme is having a salutary effect both in terms of health and literary productiveness.[14]

Day five continues to implicate the voice of medical authority in the narrator's scheme. The opening prose offers a caustic assessment of several contemporaries, M. de Luynes and the Marquis d'Ancre, whose acts were born out of their corrupting times. This wisdom, it is soon revealed, comes to us from the mouth of the visiting doctor, "comme j'ay ouy très bien dire à un medecin, heritier en partie de la bosse et du sçavoir de son père, qui tastoit le poux de madame l'accouchée" [as I heard tell by a doctor, inheritor of both the hunched back and wisdom of his father, who was taking the pulse of the newly delivered mistress] (148). This philosophizing about corruption, love, and politics weds the voice of the medical establishment, midwives, and the narrator in telling ways. The narrator borrows this authority. The transfer of narrative authority is quick and clear. In the ensuing events, the visiting doctor offers advice on remedies for love and its consequences; a midwife violently and boisterously protests; and the narrator takes his place right where the doctor had sat and consulted:

> Sur quoy M. le medecin … print congé de l'accouchée fort humblement, avec un estonnement nom-pareil de ce que ceste garde disoit contre luy; je me mis à entretenir l'accouchée, et peu après quatre dames de qualité arrivèrent en la chambre de l'accouchée … [et] prindrent place … et moy je pris la mienne ordinaire au cabinet. (148–9)
>
> [Upon which the doctor, dumbfounded, humbly took leave of the newly delivered mother, with unparalleled astonishment at what the attendant had said against him; I then set about talking with the newly delivered mother and soon thereafter appeared four women of quality who took their places and I, my usual place as well in the closet.]

However ridiculed—and this would be the order of the day for such satire which regularly references the good doctor Rabelais—medical discourse in its various guises rules the nest, as it were. The narrator increasingly implicates himself in this parlance and in its generative possibilities.

In the following *caquets*, the set-up becomes somewhat less uniform: as the previous installments have become public and circulated among the real-life gossips of Paris, references to their renown (or notoriety) become the stuff of the publications themselves. The original pamphlets demonstrate this change in

---

[14] As the days progress, so, illogically yet symbolically, does the number of offspring. On day seven, we read: "Madame a raison, dit l'accouchée; moy qui ay sept enfans …" [My lady is right, said the newly delivered mother; I who have seven children …] (*Caquets* 209).

authorship, or at least of the narrative framework.[15] Day six in the original sequence of *caquets* (published in two separate editions that same year as *La responce aux trois Caquets de l'Accouchée* and *La responce des dames et bourgeoises de Paris au Caquet de l'Accouchée*) enters into full *querelle des femmes* mode with a lengthy manifesto for the glorification of the female sex in response to the calumny created by the scandal of the previously published *caquets*. Whether the tone of the sixth installment is taken as sincere or ironic (or a combination of both), the increasing momentum of medical discourse uniting the conditions of narrator and newly delivered cousin remains robust. It is here, we remember, that the narration brings into play the medical wisdom regarding women's humors. As the narrative voice is passed along in the seventh "visitation," the creative and the procreative impulses become aligned in a manner both stunning and precise: the narrator finally goes into labor. Tellingly, fittingly, it is not a birth so much as an afterbirth that is invoked, and the scribe is eager to convey his story and dispel its mystery.

The scribe has conceived his story by the ear and eye (two recurring allusions that will be taken up in subsequent birthing narratives), listening surely, but also a present, visual witness to the *caqueteuses*. He declares somewhat redundantly: "[C]omme tesmoin occulaire de ce que j'ay veu, je vous traceray en ces lignes ce que j'en ay apris depuis peu" [As a visual witness to what I saw, I will sketch out for you in these lines what I have recently learned] (201). His description of the product of this labor merits citation at length:

> Ce que je fais icy ce n'est qu'en forme d'ARRIERE-FAIX.
> Plusieurs s'arresteront icy sur ce mot d'arrière-faix, qui, peut-estre, n'ayant jamais penetré dans les cabinets de la medecine, ignoreront de prime-abord ce que je veux entendre par la superficie de ce discours; mais ayant visité le dedans et veu ce que j'y couche, ils verront qu'à juste tiltre je devois en ce lieu parler de l'arrière-faix de l'accouchée, puisque jusques icy on en avoit tant et tant fait de ceremonies.
>
> L'arrière-faix, si nous nous voulons rapporter à madame Perrette, sage-femme du faux-bourg Sainct-Marceau, n'est autre chose qu'une superfluité de matière qui s'esvacuë hors de la matrice après l'enfantement, laquelle superfluité, comme elle est excrementielle, aussi estant retenuë dans les concavitez de la matrice et engluée dans les membranes qui se retrouvent là dedans, cela eut de beaucoup incommodé l'accouchée; c'est pourquoy il la faut jetter dehors, afin qu'estant

[15] "Il y a plus d'un mois entier que dedans Paris on nous appelle caqueteuses; on ne parle que du caquet des femmes. Jamais le lict de l'accouchée ne fut mieux remué; il est souvent retourné et feuilletté" [For more than a full month we are known about Paris as the chatterers; the only topic of conversation is the chatter of women. Never was the childbed more agitated; it (the bed? the caquets?) are constantly turned over and leafed through] (*Caquets* 187).

> reintegrée dans sa première santé, que nous aussi, ayons l'honneur d'assister au baptesme de son enfant[.] (201–2)

> [What I am making here is but an afterbirth. Some will stumble upon this word 'afterbirth,' those who, perhaps, having never penetrated the secrets of the medical cabinet would not understand at first blush what I wish to convey even at the most superficial level by such language; but having visited the inside and seen what I am birthing, they will see that it is most appropriate that I should speak here of the afterbirth of the newly delivered mother, since we have up to this point made such a big deal of it. The afterbirth, should we rely on Madame Perrette, midwife of the faux-bourg Sainct-Marceau, is nothing more than a superfluous matter that issues from the womb after birth, which, being excremental, can also be retained in the folds of the womb and stuck to the membranes that are found therein, causing great discomfort to the newly delivered mother; this is why it must be expelled, so that once she has regained her original health, and we (I) as well, we both can have the honor of attending the christening of her child(.)]

The scribe now indulges the birthing body and its metaphors with precision and researched authority; the tone is earnest and pedagogical (or is at least an affectation thereof). As he makes allusions to the presumed medical mystery of afterbirth, he guides and assures the reader. As in a manual, his main concept is in block letters; his prose style engages our possible ignorance and will to learn: "Plusieurs s'arresteront icy sur ce mot …" and he invokes the authority of a well-known midwife from Paris to help explicate his metaphor and to connect it more closely to the panoply of women's voices that constitute the *caquets*. The choice of the midwife, Madame Perrette, as gynecological authority, is remarkable and fitting for the effect of imbuing the narrative with female experience and oversight. Indeed, the syntax at the end of this critical passage betrays again a certain slippage between his identity and that of the surrounding assembly: "qu'estant reintegrée dans sa première santé, que nous aussi, ayons l'honneur …" His cousin's health ("*sa* santé") is restored, then his in the next clause ("que *nous* aussi"); curiously, then, the "nous" transfers from him (as "royal" we) to the more literal "us": she and I, off to the christening. The health of the newly delivered mother and of the cousin are neatly collapsed. The conflation, and perhaps vague confusion, of these two actors is mirrored in the closing moments of the seventh day, as the *caqueteuses* and the narrator take their leave:

> Sur cet adieu, toutes les bourgeoises prirent congé d'elle, avec toutes sortes de reverence et de courtoisie, et moy particulierement, qui sortis le dernier, et eus le bonheur de voir l'enfant dont est question et du quel on attent le baptesme. De vous dire en ce lieu si c'est un masle ou une femelle, ce seroit trop entreprendre; j'ayme mieux attendre à la première occasion. (215)

> [With this good-bye, all of the women took their leave of her, with all manner of polite reverences, and I in particular, who left last and had the joy of seeing the child in question and whose baptism we await. To tell you here if it's a male or female would be too risky; I prefer to wait for the official announcement.]

In the context of the lengthy series of *caquets* that this enterprise has produced, this particular moment is arresting, for it is the one and only time that the child is mentioned.[16] We appear, finally, to be getting a peek at the newborn—a crucial moment at any lying-in. Our hopes are spoiled, however, as we are not even allowed to know its sex, let alone any other remarkable characteristics, the stuff that might fuel, for example, a lively round of gossip. We are cut off. The "reveal" is forestalled, and the narrator takes a certain delight in this mystery, a bit of confusion that parallels the conflation of the narrator and his cousin. He has, in the telling, crossed into her gender and, at least symbolically, delivered her afterbirth. They are intimately and profoundly co-implicated in this gesture that is at first highly revealing (the lengthy disquisition on afterbirth) and concealing: What did she actually birth? This gender slippage is also evident in a previous *caquet* in a way that may help answer this question. In the second day's *caquet*, following a discussion of the poor who seem to have overrun the city of Paris, several cacklers weigh in, one citing some official ordinances promoted by court. The narrator's rejoinder to the discussion is: "Chacun approuvoit assez son dire, quand une tavernière de l'Université se leva" [Each (masculine singular) was applauding her statement when a (female) tavern keeper from the University quarter arose] (66). As Mercier rightly notes in his edition of the second *caquet*:

> Curieux masculin que ce chacun pour un symposium de dames seules! On pourrait y voir un lapsus, une étourderie de compositeur. Mais il se trouve qu'en décrivant l'arrivée des commères chez la jeune mère, tout comme il l'avait déjà fait dans *Le Caquet de l'accouchée*, l'auteur souligne que "chacun prend sa place." Est-il rétif aux désinences féminines? Veut-il affirmer la prépondérance de sa voix? Ou bien, dans son désir d'un profond changement politique, insinue-t-il que toutes gens de bon sens, avec lui, plébiscitent impatiemment le roi rédempteur?[17]

> [Strangely masculine this "chacun" for an exclusively women's symposium! One might suspect an oversight, a certain absentmindedness on the part of the writer. But it is also true that in describing the arrival of the gossips at the young mother's home, just as he did in *Le Caquet de l'accouchée*, the author remarks

---

[16] This passage is different in the *Recueil général* so it is therefore the invention of the author of the original pamphlet only. Again, the individual pamphlets and collections go through a number of editions that add and delete for uniformity. I take this passage on its own merit as part of the original rejoinder in the succession of entries.

[17] Alain Mercier, *La Seconde après-dînée du caquet de l'accouchée*, pp. 130–31.

that "each (masculine singular) took his place." Is he so contrary to feminine endings? Does he wish to affirm the importance of his own voice? Or perhaps, in his desire for profound political change, is he implying that all people of good sense, along with him, are impatiently and overwhelmingly approving the royal redeemer?]

Scribe and squabblers, *caquet* and *caqueteuse* are sharing not only gossip but gender, it appears. Mercier also points to the "*chacun* prend sa place" (43) from earlier in the chapter as the presumably all-female assembly—which would suggest "*chacune*"—is settling in.[18] This "strangely masculine" pronoun is at the heart of my answer to what is being birthed, a question to which I return in my conclusion.

If that question remains suspended, however, clearly the narrator's does not. He has pushed out ("il faut la jetter dehors") an afterbirth, what modern French gynecology terms the "délivrance." The term refers to the membrane that surrounds the fetus as well as to the placenta, the organ that is grown for nourishment and connected to the uterine walls, allowing the exchange of oxygen and blood and the evacuation of waste through the mother's kidneys. As the sixteenth-century surgeon Ambroise Paré defines it:

> L'arriere-faix a esté ainsi appelé du vulgaire, parce qu'il vient aprés l'enfant, & qu'il est un autre fais à la femme; le lict, parce que l'enfant y est couché & envelopé, & y demeure; des autres la delivrance, parce qu'estant hors, la femme est entierement delivrée.[19]
>
> [The afterbirth was named as such in the vernacular because it came after the child and is therefore another product of the woman; the bed, because the child lies there, is enveloped by it, and lives there; deliverance, because once it is outside, the woman is completely delivered.]

Such a characterization of his work fits well with the chronology that is respected in each of the eight *caquets*: the *accouchée* and the scribe have progressed gradually from postpartum melancholy, to higher spirits ("Arrière toute melancolie!"), to this talk of afterbirth and finally, in the last installment, to the "relèvement," the end of the lying-in and the mother's re-entry into society.[20]

---

[18] To be sure the pronomial norm is feminine, as at the end of the fifth day where "chacune se retira à son enseigne" (*Caquets* 183).

[19] Ambroise Paré, *Deux livres de chirurgie* ... (Paris, 1573), p. 98.

[20] Literally speaking, the afterbirth is delivered soon after the child; for the literary purposes of the narrator, however, it makes sense to speak of his work as coming along at a slightly more protracted pace. If the narrator is going to speak of his labor as distinct from that of the mother who first births her child, his expulsion of the afterbirth with its own attendant labor and delivery, will logically come later. In the conceit of the sequestered

The Placental Text: Afterlife of an Afterbirth

Having read closely the collected version of *Les Caquets* and proposed an appreciation of these pamphlets as a narrative that evinces an ever stronger connection between the male narrator's labor of one sort and his female cousin's of another, it remains to discuss the consequences of this gendered appropriation. I suggest here, as promised earlier, a view to this text that holds a number of voices in conversation as a way of opening up new possibilities on what seem like old misogynistic quarrels.

Domna Stanton (to whom I owe the term "placental text") criticizes Bakhtin's misogynistic pose with regard to the *caquets*, taking the critic to task for his complicity in the devaluation of women's speech as "nothing but gossip and tittle-tattle."[21] She argues, "Concerned with the privatizing implications of eavesdropping on chamber intimacies, he does not consider the masculine subject position of the narrator of the *caquets*, much less examine gender ideology in scenes of recuperating women" (248). Stanton then explicates this ideology in a way that ties both the author of the *caquets* and Bakhtin to particular ideological agendas—response to the "troubled and unpopular Regency of Marie de Médicis" for the former, to Marx in the latter.

> Beyond their devaluation of women's talk, *Les Caquets de l'accouchée* recuperate the exclusive femaleness of the lying-in through the presence of the voyeuristic male narrator. By penetrating this space, he symbolically avenges the excluded male … In this phantasmatic ambiance, the cackling woman at the lying-in may function as the ludicrous correlative of Marie, the maternal virago; in the phallic imaginary, women's license—discursive and/as political—threatens male rules(s). Far from being a trivially private text, as Bakhtin claims, the male-narrated *Recueil général des caquets de l'accouchée* recuperates the "loose talk" of women at the lying-in, and then uses it as a screen to denounce social disorder and to proclaim the cure of rigid, patriarchal rule. (250, 251)

Fears of women monarchs, of birthing bodies, and of women's gossip converge for Stanton in this vexing text. Crucial to her argument is the newly delivered woman's acceptance of her objectification and her status as the narrator's alibi. She "assuages men's phantasmatic fear of—and repulsion from—the fertile maternal body at the birth-giving scene" (253). Thus, Stanton reads the afterbirth reference

---

scribe whose matter—here the afterbirth—is nourished and produced by gossip, one must wait at least some time for the cackling to be transcribed and delivered.

[21] Domna C. Stanton, "Recuperating Women and the Man behind the Screen," in James Grantham Turner (ed.), *Sexuality and Gender in Early Modern Europe: Institutions, Texts, Images* (Cambridge, 1993), p. 247. Quotations from Bakhtin here and in her article are from Mikhail Bakhtin, *Rabelais and His World*, trans. Hélène Iswolsky (Bloomington, 1984), pp. 105–6.

as utterly and entirely derisive, taking this consummately Rabelaisian excremental issuance as a keenly misogynistic gesture: birth and afterbirth; coveted progeny and vile waste, the one folded into the other as the narrator's plan foils and fouls women's procreative capacity.

Stanton's term "recuperating women" plays with recuperation on three levels simultaneously: as the process of regaining one's health; as the nefarious narrator's appropriation and defilement of the woman's body; and, in the end, as a call for a feminist reassessment and revalorization of women's discourse by the example of the *caquets*' most earthy, radical, and regenerative rejoinders, *Les Essais de Mathurine*, contained in the *Recueil général*. Mathurine was an actual personnage of humble origins who was sheltered in the court of Marie de Médicis as a "folle du logis" [female jester], dispensing unfiltered observations on all who crossed her path.[22] The text attributed to her is, to follow Stanton's term, a recuperation of women's right to assemble and cackle. According to Stanton, and I would concur, Mathurine's text far outstrips its predecessor in the contest of Rabelaisian wit. Stanton praises the Mathurine intervention as follows: "Affirming female sexuality and her own *jouissance*, Mathurine traces the narrator/author's contempt for women to the hideous old whore who promised him great potency … but who gave him, instead, a venereal 'love sickness'" (260). It is Mathurine's scatalogical retorts concerning the scribe's own conception and birth that most interest me here. Deriding the very concept of a *caqueteux*, or male gossip, she drags him through a birthing body in the most excremental of ways:

> Quiconque fait le caqueteux, jamais bonne pie ne le couva, et la semence de quoy il fust basti estoit esvantée aussi bien que sa cervelle. Peut-estre eust-il rongé, ainsi que comme les vipereaux, le ventre de sa mère pour sortir, s'il ne se fust trouvé vers la basse cartière une bonde grandement large; et, parcequ'elle luy fit baiser son cul en passant, qui estoit un peu sale pour lors, et deceda sans hoirs legitimes de son corps, il voudroit prendre à tasche tout le sexe féminin. (*Caquets* 253–4)
>
> [Whosoever plays the male gossip (cackler), no good magpie (chatterbox) would ever have brooded over him, and the seed that made him would have been spoiled, just like his brains. Perhaps he would have gnawed through the belly of his mother to get out as vipers do, had he not found a sufficiently large gate in her nether regions; and, because she made him kiss her ass on his way out, which was a bit dirty at the time, and died without a legitimate heir from her body, he wants to despoil the entire female sex.]

This is indeed a very powerful "recuperation" of women's generative and degenerative power, fueling all manner of fears of women's bodies as polluted, uncontrolled, toxic, and bestial. Her womb becomes a viper's nest and the narrator

---

22 See the Le Roux de Lincy edition of the *caquets*, p. xxiii.

is its inhuman—because unwelcome and unnatural—resident: he has penetrated the "womb" of his cousin's *ruelle* and been hideously transformed for it. Mathurine, thus, re-recuperates the sanctum of the lying-in and the birthing body, throwing it back at the presumptuous narrator, laughing all the way. The kind of birthing in which the impertinent (and here construed as illegitimate) *caqueteux* can participate can only be foul and morbid: he and his text are thoroughly debased and degraded, allied as they are with disease, uncertain paternity and, perhaps most importantly, matricide—the devouring of the very vessel and process he has attempted to appropriate.

The work of Gianna Pomata in Finucci and Brownlee's influential volume of essays, *Generation and Degeneration: Tropes of Reproduction in Literature and History*, informs this discussion in a way that rather turns the propensity to demonize the female reproductive body on its head. Pomata's revolutionary thesis regarding early modern assessments of women's bodily functions is allied to such thoroughgoing investigation of a vast corpus of medical literature from the period that one cannot help but welcome her important work into the conversation. What might menstruating men and birthing men have to say to each other?

Pomata's essay, "Menstruating Men: Similarity and Difference of the Sexes in Early Modern Medicine," recuperates the menstruating body as normative and healthy within the discourses of early modern European medicine.[23] By reviewing numerous cases of periodic bleeding interpreted as "vicarious menstruation" (110), Pomata challenges notions of the primacy of the male body as superior. "Our notion of menstruation as a specifically female trait stands in stark contrast with these descriptions of menstruating men. These stories clearly imply perceptions of what is male and female that differ from ours in one of its most basic tenets" (112). The basic tenet is that of the one-sexed, male-normative body, promoted most radically by Thomas Laqueur's study, *Making Sex*. While she does not contest that there was a clear emphasis on the similarity of the sexes, Pomata proposes the novel idea that, based on the stories of menstruating men, the female body was the *Gestalt*. Her menstruating body was cleansing, purgative, salutary, and indeed medically desirable. Pomata's approach to the fascinating fund of case studies which come to us through the traditions of *curatio* (narratives of the unfolding of a disease from onset to cure) and *observatio* (the reporting of natural events in general) privilege the genre first and foremost as a good story (114), whence their added pertinence to *Les Caquets de l'accouchée*, whose narrator, as I have attempted to show, prizes both medical knowledge and a good read.

Of particular interest is Pomata's framing and presentation of the *observatio* by Simon Schultz in the *Ephemerides* of the *Academia Naturae Curiosorum*, penned a bit later in the seventeenth century. I quote at length for the number of associations that both she and Schultz provide:

---

[23] Gianna Pomata, "Menstruating Men: Similarity and Difference of the Sexes in Early Modern Medicine," in Valeria Finucci and Kevin Brownlee (eds), *Generation and Degeneration: Tropes of Reproduction in Literature and History* (Durham, NC, 2001).

These are often stories that the doctors learnt from having intimately known the menstruating men as personal friends rather than patients. Some of these stories appear to be based on confidential disclosures from man to man about a peculiar experience that cut across social distinctions (the cases reported concern men of every social class—beggars and peasants as well as patricians and intellectuals). Intimate male gossip, we might call it, clad in the dignified garb of medical observation. Take as one more example this story from the *Ephemerides* of 1684:

The nobleman Felix Rauschart, counselor to the duke of Saxony and a most honored friend of mine, a man of sanguine and melancholic complexion … was affected for the first time with hemorrhoidal flow. Nature has ever since regularly repeated this flux every month up to the present day … It should be noted that every time the hemorrhoidal discharge is irregular either in time or quantity, his natural faculties appear to be disturbed and weakened in consequence: namely, he is afflicted by constipation, difficulty in breathing, inflammation of the hypochondrium accompanied by general exhaustion of body and soul. As soon as the flow comes back all these symptoms disappear. (Pomata 117)

Les Caquets de l'accouchée are nothing if not intimate male gossip (female *caquets* filtered through the male narrator) clad in the dignified garb of medical observation. In Pomata's examples, the curious tales of menstruating men are conveyed from man to man but then displayed for a reading public thirsty for such curiosities. The ways in which the doctor reports the transcendence of class and station is also germane to the discussion of *Les Caquets*, wherein the author(s) make a point of including women and topics of discussion from throughout the social spectrum—a facet of the narrative that is quite pertinent to my conclusion. Furthermore, the men in question languish and are melancholic when their regular cycles are interrupted. The general exhaustion of body and soul is not far from the description that our narrator conveys at the beginning of *Les Caquets*; his "flow" as it were—the ejection of his afterbirth—has yet to occur and he is, as the Galenic paradigms of plethora might imply, overwhelmed and unpurged, awaiting the expulsion of his corrupted humors—a medical allusion that he makes clear, as we have already seen (*Caquets* 133). And expulsion leads always to positive outcomes in the stories that Pomata so privileges:

Let us look at the stories of menstruating men or of the menses "unusual pathways" simply as stories, stories with an ending. They are all—either when intended to prove the theory of plethora or that of fermentation—stories with a happy ending: examples of longevity, fertility, or recovery. (Pomata 136)

To be clear, Pomata does not dispute the ambient Aristotelian assumptions about the superiority of the male body; she recuperates, however, the optimal qualities evidenced in women's *menses*, a condition that medical practice—through leeching and bloodletting, for example, and through positive associations with other evidence of bleeding (hemorrhoids and nosebleeding)—amply confirms (134).

To conclude my appreciation of Pomata's hopeful and feminist assessment of this rather bizarre, albeit seemingly common and amply documented medical phenomenon, I cite her explication of another briefly presented case whose particulars are not needed here; the case could be like any of the many she cites wherein men's health is restored through what is characterized as menstruation:

> What we see here is a man whose perception of his own body is deeply influenced by the model of female physiology. The periodic flux of blood that gives him relief is something that he perceives as part of his normal condition: "a regular and ordinary aspect of nature," as he calls it—of his own nature, not just that of women. A female conception of nature, as we see, may have very important consequences, theoretical as well as practical. (141)

My hope here is to see *Les Caquets*, given the scribe's willingness to medicalize and dramatize his own *curatio*, as it were, as participating, wittingly or not, in a view to women's bodies, even parodically, that is generative, restorative, and salutary. He has been purged; he has expulsed; and his story is based in, on, and about the secrets and marvels of the birthing body, as richly Rabelaisian as he wishes to make it. Finally, as Pomata observes, "In this conception of the healing process, the abstract entity 'nature' was identified with something very specific in deed: the lowest and humblest among bodily processes, the body's excretory function. The body—but which body? It was the female body that was the primary model of nature's healing" (138). Both the anonymous scribe's "placental text" and Mathurine's scatological and bestial births might, therefore, be recuperated into a powerful female, dare one say feminist, reappraisal of the creative and procreative woman's body. Stanton admonishes Bakhtin for participating in the dismissal of the *Les Caquets* as "tittle-tattle" and hopes to reappropriate the value of women's speech, mainly by pulling Mathurine into the discussion—a gesture I hope to have furthered along in my reading. But with the help of Pomata's work, I have tried to push even further and implicate the scribe as well as participating in a paradigm of labor, birthing, lying-in, and re-entry into society in a way that also values women's procreative potential. He has played the medical authority card; he has assumed the status of the laboring woman; he has "birthed" a bizarre yet highly popular and widely published "text." It seems not unproductive to take him at his word. It remains to be seen what he actually delivered and how this might be construed in the context of seventeenth-century literary society.

A Prehistory of the *Ruelles*?

I began this chapter by looking back to the literary precedent that informed the misogynistic literary genre, as it were, of cackling women and beleaguered men from previous centuries. I shift in this final section to a view of *Les Caquets* as precedent itself to the literary milieu of the salon and all of the antifeminist energy to which it may have responded. The recovering scribe's refuge in the *ruelle* seems too suggestive to leave uninvestigated. To this end, I now focus more closely on how the voice of the narrator is constructed and in what company this voice of authority claims to be speaking. The scribe at the lying-in has textually transgendered himself into a community of women that "cackle" about a range of literary and social events, drawing conspicuous attention to a privileged bedside *côterie* with a range of insights and viewpoints on current events and contemporary attitudes in the Paris of 1622. Can Rambouillet's *chambre bleue*, inaugurated over a decade before, be far from the reader's imagination? I begin with a brief return to the way in which the propitious and (re)productive lying-in is conceived.

If we noticed an intriguing slippage in the narrator's gendering of the assembled *caqueteuses*—"*chacun* prend sa place, *chacun* approuvoit assez son dire" (emphasis mine)—so does the voice of the scribe shift between male and female, revealing a hybrid, collaborative text with multiple, at times competing subject positions that are woven into the collected work. In reinvestigating this text, I propose a view to this society as often multi-gendered (as the salon would be), a slippage or slip of a Freudian cast: while the familiar conceit in *Les Caquets* is one of gossiping women, the contemporary influence of other less gender-exclusive societies overwhelms it. Genre and gender alike become necessarily fluid and confused as the text accommodates the denizens of the *ruelle*. So, as the narrator appropriates for himself the reproductive capacities of his cousin during her confinement, so might he be appropriating, redefining, and perhaps parodying a budding literary and political milieu increasingly recognizable to seventeenth-century society. The anonymous and often ambiguous status of the narrator over the successive installments suggests this with increasing insistence.

The first five pamphlets of *Les Caquets* are in the voice of a male narrator, who, as we have seen, evolves through progressively less melancholic states. The story of the visiting cousin is maintained here and the frame narrative is given a fair bit of attention—over a fourth of the total text in the first and fifth days.[24] In the preparatory prose to day four, the narrator exclaims:

> [N]ous nous entretinsmes long-temps des discours facetieux qui s'estoient faits à notre dernière entreveuë, de la deffiance des dames, du conte que l'on leur avoit fait que quelqu'un se cachoit en la ruelle du lict, et mesme de leur curieuse recherche. Nous en rismes à gorge desployée. Elle s'informa des nouvelles du Palais … (*Caquets* 118)

---

[24] I arrive at this approximate percentage by counting lines devoted to the set-up of the day's *caquet* as compared to the interventions by the visiting women.

> [We compared notes at length about the mischievous tales that were cooked up at our last session, about the mistrust of the women and about the story one had told them of someone hiding in the space between the bed and the wall and even about their silly searching about. We laughed wholeheartedly about that. She then asked about news from the Palais …]

The cousins have their private moments, then, where they go back over their ruse and thrill to the near discovery of their plan and the deception of their gossiping guests. But as the passage shows, they soon tumble into their own version of *caqueterie* as she inquires about affairs at court and is regaled with a tale of cuckoldry and spying, not unlike the very situation that they have created for themselves.

The sixth day is a clear departure from the scenario, at least as presented in the original pamphlet. This installment, *La responce des dames et bourgeoises de Paris au Caquet de l'Accouchée*, is signed by Mademoiselle E. D. M. The frame of the *ruelle* in this original is decidedly not respected here—quite the opposite:

> Comme je fus arrivée aux baings où d'ordinaire nous avons coustume entre nous autres de nous rafraichir, je me trouvay au milieu d'une bonne et agreable compaignie de bourgeoises et dames de Paris. (186)

> [As I arrived at the baths where ordinarily we would cool off amongst ourselves, I found myself in the midst of the good and pleasurable company of women and ladies of Paris.]

The female assembly then disrobes, glides into the water, and considers its plight as played out in the notorious *caquets*. In the original, then, this is an insider's view, *entre nous*. There is no deception and the response is a rendering of events and conversation as told by one of their own. Their day of bathing and commiserating terminates in a group letter of protest, disavowing the monstrous *caquets* that have so sullied their reputation. And with that, they depart:

> De là, s'estant toutes revestues, elles sortirent des estuves et s'en retournèrent chacune en son logis, avec promesse toutefois de s'assembler pour la seconde et troisième fois, si l'occasion le requiert. (200)

> [Therewith, having gotten dressed again, they left the steam baths and returned each to her own house, promising to reassemble for a second or third time should circumstances require it.]

The attention to their re-dressing reminds the reader of their previous nakedness and the very private, feminine gathering that has occurred. And they are united: they have penned their manifesto and dedicated themselves to solidarity and future meetings of support as conditions should require.

The seventh day is the pivotal moment in which the narrator takes on most viscerally the corporeal metaphor of the birthing body, with his lesson on early modern gynecology and his text become afterbirth. The narrative voice, as bizarrely connected to female anatomy as it is, is male, and his entry into his cousin's chamber is curiously thwarted. She is now up and about and the narrator has already had a furtive peek at her through a crack in the door as she was attending to her *toilette*. Disguised as an apothecary, he gains entry with the other women callers later in the day. He has painted himself as the jilted lover or cuckolded husband and plays along, disguises and all. In the final day, there is still some conceit of a male narrator, but he is clearly slipping away. After some lofty opening rhetoric he is invoked in the third person and again in a way that links him to his cousin's postpartum condition:

> Excusons-le, il est sur l'aage, il est chargé de beaucoup d'enfans, et sur tout d'une grande fille qui ne peut trouver un bon party faute d'escus; et puis il est nouvellement relevé de maladie … (218)
>
> [Let us excuse him, he's getting on in years, he's loaded down with children, and most of all by an older daughter who can't find a good suitor for lack of money; and in addition, he is just recovered from an illness …]

Here the line between the cousins' identities is very flimsy, and comically so. The portrait of the narrator, surrounded by multiple children and newly recovering from illness (described, as we have seen, as postpartum melancholy), is certainly that of a *mother*, not father, however beleaguered he might feel at the demands of a sufficient dowry. The first person does eventually appear, but without connection to the frame story; he and his cousin do not speak to each other and the interventions of the women attendants surface as if from nowhere, responding without any arrival or context having been given. Fittingly, the *caqueteuses* and the narrator trail off into silence. A servant brings them strong drink and implores them to stop cackling about lovemaking and get to it:

> Par ma foy, il vaut mieux n'en guères dire et en faire davantage. Çà, çà, beuvons le temps le permet, et puis nos maris n'y sont pas. Ce qui donna tant de hardiesse à la compagnie, qu'aussi tost les dames commencèrent d'escrimer du gobelet et d'articuler des machoires à bon esceint, observant chascune d'elles un silence nompareil. (235)
>
> [Good gracious, it's better to stop talking about it and rather have at it. There, there, let's drink in the time that remains, and now that our husbands are not here. This got the group quite fired up so much so that they began clinking their goblets and working their jaws, so that an unaccustomed silence was observed.]

It is a fittingly Rabelaisian ending, echoing the newborn Gargantua's "A boire! A boire!" and that author's indebtedness to drink in the same tale's prologue. This is followed by the dramatic effect of silence, the antithesis of cackling. The mouths of the gossips are finally corked; the pen of the scribe is stilled: the end of the lying-in (the cousin's *relèvement*) signals the end of stories and the completion of the *caquets*, both literal and literary, with the caveat in the *Recueil* that they part ways, "se promettant les unes aux autres, d'un vif courage, de se voir à leurs autres accouchemens" [promising each other quite assuredly to meet up again at future births] (235).

Having begun this exploration of *Les Caquets de l'accouchée* by reviewing its literary precedents in the female-defined *Les Quinze joies de mariage* and the *Les Evangiles des quenouilles* and paid close attention to the two principal characters in this literary conceit (the postpartum cousins), I propose a reading of this phenomenon as a nascent critique of Parisian salon culture, a milieu defined by women, established at the bedside, and altogether engaged in the literary culture of its day. The narrator's plot as directed by his doctor is to "glisser *à la ruelle du lict* une apresdinée pour entrendre les nouvelles" [slip *into the space beside her bed* after dinner to hear the stories] and the patient complies, asking his cousin in exactly this language "de me cacher à la ruelle du lict aux apresdinées, pour entendre le discours des femmes" [to hide me in the space beside the bed after dinner to hear the women talking]. As we have seen, the terminology changes over the course of the successive installments—he refers to his *cabinet* and *études* at various moments—but the *ruelle* remains constant, both within the individual pamphlets and in the *Recueil*. A *ruelle* then, is the privileged space in which the anonymous narrator takes up his pen, listening, recording, and, at times, going over the events with his cousin after the society has dispersed, proud of his burgeoning register of gossip.

While the dates for the first usage of the term *ruelle* as a literary milieu are not precise, it is entirely conceivable that by 1622 this was a deliberate reference. As we shall see, salon scholar Faith Beasley agrees with conventional acceptance of Madame de Rambouillet's *chambre bleue* as the advent of the seventeenth-century salon as defined by the *ruelle*—the first *salonnière* to receive in bed. Beasley concurs with Linda Timmermans regarding the suggestion of even earlier proto-salons hosted by the vicontesse d'Auchy and Madame des Loges. Madeleine and Catherine des Roches, of course, entertained a large *côterie* of socially and literarily prominent men and women toward the end of the preceding century.[25] I propose a reading of this company and its criticism—suggested through the misogyny both within the text and in its redaction over time—as participating in an anxiety about

[25] See Linda Timmermans, *L'Accès des femmes à la culture (1598–1715)* (Paris, 1993), pp. 71–84. For the Des Roches, see Anne R. Larsen, *From Mother and Daughter: poems, dialogues, and letters of les dames des Roches/Madeleine and Catherine des Roches* (Chicago, 2006), "Introduction."

women's collaborative speech and assembly in the early seventeenth century. To this end, we should look a bit further into the assembly and what they were up to.

If *Les Quinze joies de mariage* and *Les Evangiles des quenouilles* exploit cuckoldry as their basic theme, with some folk wisdom and social commentary thrown in on the side, *Les Caquets de l'accouchée* (while not unconcerned with philandering spouses) presents a far more wide-ranging array of topics with, by comparison, an enormous cast of characters from all walks of life. Cuckoldry and spying provide a seductive tension that inflects this rarified milieu, but this docs not determine it. On the contrary, more remarkable is the variety in the themes and in the cast of characters:

> [A]rrivèrent, de toutes parts, toutes sortes de belles dames, damoiselles, jeunes, vieilles, riches et médiocres, de toutes façons, qui, après avoir faict le salut ordinaire, prindrent place chacun selon son rang et dignité, puis commencèrent à caqueter comme il s'ensuit … (*Caquets* 12)
>
> [They arrived, from all over, all sorts of fine women, ladies, girls, old women, rich and of modest means, of all sorts, who, after the perfunctory salutations, took their place according to their rank and station, and began to gossip as follows …]

As Alain Mercier reports in his edition of the *Seconde après-dînée de l'accouchée*, no fewer than 76 interlocutors grace the presence of the newly delivered cousin. While many of those in attendance are only summarily identified ("une Rousse du mesme cartier," etc.) fully half are described with fair attention to their social standing: seven ladies of the aristocracy; 13 officers' wives of middle or high standing; two unmarried "bourgeoises;" two middle-class wives identified by their husbands' public service; two merchants' wives; the wife of a university astrologer; seven vendors of modest social standing; a sculptor; a midwife, and two domestic servants (Mercier 127–8). And from this variety of voices emerges a witty and irreverent commentary on the events of the day—a window onto the scandals and controversies of Parisian society in 1622. From Mercier's commentary on the second day only:

> L'actualité récente inspire l'essentiel des caquets. C'est d'abord la lutte contre les factions protestantes, l'action militaire, tactique et diplomatique du gouvernement pour juguler ces fiefs de la révolte; l'attitude des hommes politiques dans cette croisade qui exacerbe les passions … Chronique savoureuse des temps d'incertitude, *La Seconde Apres-disnee* se lit comme une page d'Histoire pleine d'humour, de colère et d'espoir. C'est le manifeste d'un homme talentueux, à la plume alerte et inventive. (129–30)

> [The core of the *caquets* is inspired by current events. Primarily the struggle against the Protestant factions, military maneuvers, governmental tactics, and diplomacy regarding the control of revolting fiefdoms; the attitude of crusading politicians in the heat of passion. A sumptuous chronicle of a time of great uncertainty, *La Seconde Apres-disnee* reads like a page torn from History, full of humor, anger, and hope. It is the manifesto of a talented man, possessed of a lively and inventive wit.]

Religion, military action, and economic policy (including discussions of plans that resemble nothing so much as economic stimulus packages) bubble alongside questions of infidelity, pretense, appearances, sumptuary laws, and social standing. While much is made of the salacious and scatological nature of *Les Caquets*, the subject of the cackling is inspired far more by contemporary events. As Domna Stanton rightly points out, "the theme of sexuality in *Les Caquets* pales by comparison with the depiction of social corruption that dominates the women's gossip. Money, far more than sex, makes the world go round in the words of these predominantly bourgeois, but also upper- and lower-class, women, who cite names and places that create 'libellous' *effets de reel*." (Stanton 256).

And all along—and ever more obviously toward the end of the *Recueil*—the subject of literature and of the literary phenomenon of *Les Caquets* itself becomes the topic of conversation. In the third *caquet*, a councilor's wife bemoans:

> [O]n fit present l'autre jour à mon mary d'un petit discours intitulé l'Esprit de la Cour qui va de nuict; mais d'autant que la matière ne respond en façon du monde au titre, je voudrois que celui qui l'a faict eust un esprit de jour, et non pas de nuict, obscur et perdu, afin qu'il peust recognoistre ce qu'il veut escrire, car on n'y cognoist rien. (*Caquets* 106–7)

> [The other day my husband was presented with a little book entitled *l'Esprit de la Cour qui va de nuict*; but inasmuch as the content has nothing to do with the title, I would prefer that he who wrote it have a bit more *esprit de jour*, and not *de nuit*, obscure and lost as it is, so that he could recognize what he wants to write about, because one can understand nothing in it.]

While the book comes to her through her husband, she has still read it and had opinions, ideas that she finally shares in this *côterie* of women and that stimulate further discussion on misguided authors and their works. Such scrutiny is prepared in the second *caquet*, wherein the wife of a bookseller weighs in on sloppy copy editing: "on rapporta l'autre jour un livre à mon mary, où il y avoit autant de fautes que de mots" [The other day my husband was given a book where there were as many typographical errors as there were words] (46). One has the idea throughout *Les Caquets* that a number of these women are readers, consumers of literature that they critique with knowledge and great abandon. Fittingly, the fourth day ends with a lament over printers and their occasional scams. Thus, the lively discussion of the printed life is trotted out and critiqued from every angle. As we have stated, the final installments of *Les Caquets* become ever more conscious of the texts in circulation that critique, malign, and comment upon their very community—Mathurine being the most strident defender against a host of attackers.

Embedded along with these important references to the contemporary literary scene is, additionally, a critique of women's participation in such endeavors. On day two, an exchange between two crippled interlocutors (a hunchback and a clubfoot) elicits, "Mais est-ce à faire aux femmes à lire et manier un livre si hazardeux, qui tuë et occist ceux qui le veulent expliquer et manier trop indescrettement?" [But is it women's business to read and engage with such a hazardous book that kills and does in those who seek to explicate and interpret too indiscreetly?] (49) In the second day, an old woman rails on for several pages against the ills of the reformed church and then curiously self-abnegates by concluding:

> Ce n'est pas, dit-elle, aux femmes à s'entremesler si avant dans les affaires, et principalement où il s'agit de religion: car, outre que notre sexe est imbécille à proposer les raisons de part et d'autre, nous nous laissons incontinent emporter à la colère. (82)
>
> [It is not for women, said she, to get so mixed up in such affairs, and especially where religion is concerned: for, beyond the fact that our sex is utterly incapable of proposing solutions of one sort or another, we also let ourselves be transported by anger.]

She undermines her authority on the one hand, while demonstrating a passionate and well-informed critique on the other: a vigorous debate worthy of the most lively *ruelle*. Finally, in the third day, as we have seen, the newly delivered cousin expresses a desire to leave the discussion of court clerks and their livelihood to men, redirecting their attention, however, to more literary pursuits: "[C]'est à faire aux hommes de le debattre … Parlons, s'il vous plaist, d'autres choses. N'avez-vous veu et leu les questions de Tabarin?" [That is for men to debate. Let's speak, if you please, of other things. Have you not seen and read Tabarin's questions?] (93)

To characterize the authorship and the genre of *Les Caquets de l'accouchée* is, decidedly, not an easy task. Its clearest defining characteristics are its hybridity; its preoccupation with the birthing body and its attendants as a structuring mechanism—a female-defined milieu; and its indulgence of self-critique: multiple voices of both genders as subjects and objects of discourse. The lying-in chamber is, in many ways, imbued with the stuff of salon culture. It seems not a long leap from *caqueteuse* to *précieuse*—from the *ruelle* of the melancholic narrator's cousin to that of Catherine de Vivonne, marquise de Rambouillet—and perhaps fruitful to explore how *Les Caquets* not only responds to the past but also prepares the debates over women's participation in literary production and critique under way in the early seventeenth century.

Given the characterization of the subject matter of *Les Caquets* by Mercier and others, the question of history as it may be constructed in these texts demands consideration. This is a curious document in terms of a chronicle of contemporary society on a large and small scale. This "chronique savoureuse" and "Histoire pleine d'humour, de colère et d'espoir" denotes an innovative genre, as it were, born of a most innovative setting. This chronicle issued from the *ruelle* is itself marginal, or better, intermediary, defining a *ruelle* of its own, between the intimacy of sequestered gripes and confidences and a public critique of real actors in the daily life of finance, labor, religion, and government in contemporary Parisian society. At times a sort of *roman à clef*, featuring thinly veiled exposés of financial or court conspirators, and often explicit in the naming of names (the indexes to the nineteenth-century editions provide a virtual who's who of Parisian elites in 1622), *Les Caquets* participates in what Faith Beasley might term "particular history," a version of events informed by the human details of less official accountings of court and society. Beasley defines particular history in contrast with "Histoire" or general history seen as retellings of recognizable, verifiable political events in the public sector:

> Particular history seeks to reveal the details and reasoning that underlie the public matters of general history, the motives and passions that determine officially recorded events, and it includes, in addition, actions that are excluded from the general record. "Particular history," however, is not synonymous with what modern historians call "private history" because, as will become clear when we turn to the texts of particular history, the content of this account is not severed completely from that of general history or from the public sphere—a severance connoted by the term "private."[26]

To be sure, Beasley's taxonomy of historical approaches and genres privileges women's memoirs and novels as the vehicles of this brand of history; my evocation of her definition, however, is wedded to a notion of literary society that is similarly evinced in *Les Caquets*. The melancholic scribe thrives in an intentional, female-defined space and produces a text that is utterly collaborative. He and his cousin create a parallel and particular account of contemporary society together: she, providing the *ruelle*, a fair amount of personal wisdom, and the unwitting company; and he, the product of this "labor," culled from both the ruminations of the *caqueteuses* and from his very own conversations and commentaries with the cousin as they frame and nourish this enterprise. As we have remarked in the *caquets*' pronomial slippage, there is evidence to suggest that the author, at least subconsciously, envisioned a mixed-gender society akin to the constituency of, say, the *chambre bleue*, where men and women conversed, critiqued, and created together. Of even more nefarious influence perhaps, is the wholesale

[26] Faith Beasley, *Revising Memory: Women's Fiction and Memoirs in Seventeenth-Century France* (New Brunswick, 1990), p. 29.

recharacterization in the serialization of the sixth installment, whose ultimately unsuccessful appropriation of the feminist diatribe of the bathing women is subsumed into the conceit of the male malingerer/scribe: the editors of the *Recueil* do little to retrofit this decidedly female defense against the *caquets* in circulation; the messiness of this hybrid text may even more accurately mirror the polyvocality of the salon. In addition, their conversation often turns back onto the subject of their own enterprise: books, printing, editing, reviewing, and the previous installments of the *caquets* themselves becoming the stuff of their daily conversation. Finally, in response to Beasley's notion of severance, the scribe and his text are not, in my reading, cut off from official accounts of history: his plan of recovery is a ruse to, in fact, re-enter society and its intrigues. This is a collaborative, self-critiquing society of *ruelle* habitués whose sequestered, creative enterprise is hidden in plain sight and then made public by its most envious member, who assumes his host's gendered lot and makes of it the engine of his hybrid, transgressive, literary, and historical rumination.

Beasley's subsequent work on the salon also invites us to make the link between *caquetuese* and *précieuse* more consciously. She says, "Today seventeenth-century salons are synonymous with *précieuse* (precious) a term that is itself conflated not with culture but with ridicule due largely to Molière's satirical portraits of the women who frequented the salon milieu."[27] *Les Caquets* participates in grand style in this satire of society and in particular of women as cacklers and arbiters. To be sure, we are decades before the time when Molière's portraits gain traction and general currency. Nonetheless, the society that surfaces in *Les Caquets* can be read as not unlike the literary milieu that Beasley attempts to recuperate and revise. She states:

> To judge from many of the myths and histories surrounding the salons, especially the *chambre bleue*, one might be tempted to view the worldly public as diametrically opposed to the *doctes* and their academic norms, in particular to the illustrious, state-sanctioned French Academy. While their values may have differed, their habitués were the same. In reality the two spheres were enmeshed in each other, leading to a dynamic, but very complicated literary scene (*Salons* 24).

Enmeshed and complicated makes for a good description of what *Les Caquets* and its panoply of participants are all about.

The parodic nature of *Les Caquets de l'accouchée* as well as its rather maladroit redaction which, as we have seen, attempts unsuccessfully—perhaps because half-heartedly?—to homogenize its authorship, make it a difficult text to characterize in terms of salon politics. There is, admittedly, no direct reference to a specific *ruelle*, though I find the very reference, the *ruelle*-ness of this text, significant.

---

[27] Faith Beasley, *Salons, History, and the Creation of Seventeenth-Century France: Mastering Memory* (Aldershot, 2006), p. 2.

If *Les Evangiles des quenouilles* and *Les Quinze joies de mariage* strive to turn women's intercourse into cackling and malevolent gossip, so does *Les Caquets de l'accouchée* prepare the misogynistic leap from pre-Molière *salonnière* to post-Molière *précieuse*. As such, *Les Caquets* is situated within a continuum of representations of feminine community at once suspicious of, in the thrall of, and imbued with a gynocentric literary universe. As the cousin rises from childbed, one wonders for what society her *relèvement* has prepared her. It seems right and fair to give back the voice of the female narrator in the purloined sixth *caquets* and it seems long past due to reevaluate the literary value of the salon as so trenchantly established by Beasley. While the narrative voice of much of the series remains clearly male, the collaborative conceit implicates a much larger, mixed-gender production in the making. In fact, the narrator's *relèvement*, his emergence from the *ruelle*, can be seen to suggest a personal birthing of sorts: the *ruelle* become womb—a womb of his/their own (with thanks and apology to Virginia Woolf)—that affords him/them immense public influence (though anonymous) and a voice in the literary landscape of the Paris of 1622. I hope here to have situated *Les Caquets* in a literary history both beholden to misogynist portrayals of women's voice and yet potentially celebratory of a concomitant strain of collaborative production.

Afterword on Afterbirth

By way of conclusion, I return to the curious gynecological specificity of the seventh *caquet*—the afterbirth episode—to discover what is at stake not only literarily but literally for men and for women engaged as they may be in the vicissitudes of the birthing body. Royal surgeon Jacques Guillemeau, in his manual on childbirth and women's health (*De l'Heureux accouchement des femmes...* of 1609), speaks of the afterbirth in a way reminiscent of *Les Caquets*' rather paternal, pedantic tone. The afterbirth is spoken of as a potentially fatal element in the safe and successful delivery of a woman:

> Il peut arriver apres que la mere aura accouché naturellement ... que le lict sur lequel respose l'enfant (appellé vulgairement arrierefais comme estant second fais ou fardeau de la mere, ou delivre, parce qu'estant sorty, la mere est du tout delivree) demeurera attaché aux paroys de la matrice, sans se pouvoir facilement separer.[28]

> [It can happen that after the mother has given birth naturally ... that the "bed" upon which the child rests (known commonly as afterbirth being a second act

[28] Jacques Guillemeau, *De l'Heureux accouchement des femmes où il est traicté du gouvernement de leur grossesse, de leur travail naturel et contre nature, du traictement estant accouchées et de leurs maladies* (Paris, 1609), p. 313.

> or burden for the mother, or delivery, because, once out, the mother is delivered of everything) will remain attached to the wall of the uterus, unable to separate easily.]

Guillemeau cites dryness, swelling, cessation of contractions, and severe fatigue as common causes for this condition. But the delivery of the afterbirth is crucial:

> Or c'est chose certaine, qu'apres que l'enfant est sorty du ventre de la mere, que ledit arrierefais est chose contre nature, qui ne requiert sinon que d'estre osté & mis dehors, parquoy il faut de deux choses l'une, ou que le vif (qui est la matrice) chasse le mort (qui est l'arrierefais) ou que le mort tue le vif. (314)
>
> [Therefore one thing is certain, that after the child has left the mother's belly, the afterbirth is a thing against nature which requires only to be taken away and put outside, which means one of two things: either the living (which is the womb) chases away the dead (which is the afterbirth) or the dead will kill the living.]

What follows is 10 pages of medical observation and advice about how to gently extract the afterbirth. The author advises patience combined with immediate and persistent attention while the woman's body is still in flux; the mother should take a bit of soup if she is feeling weak; sneezing might be induced to help expulsion; various medicines can be concocted and ingested (the recipes are included); should manual extraction be necessary, he recommends great care of the surgeon's hands and proper lubrication; liniments and injections may be implicated; extreme care so as not to rupture, tear, or otherwise compromise the postpartum body is repeatedly advised. Remarkable in its comprehensiveness and in the delicacy with which Guillemeau insists that the potions and procedures be administered, the chapter is a riveting testimony to the potential dangers of this recalcitrant organ. This life-giving, nourishing, and sustaining "bed" upon which the infant takes succor becomes suddenly "against nature" if not expulsed. This explanation, which could easily have served as the intertext for the scribe sequestered in the *ruelle*, is a curious choice of metaphors for a man birthing a text. By the narrator's own reckoning it is "excrementielle," a "superfluité de matière" at risk of being stuck in the postpartum body—"retenuë dans les concavitez de la matrice et engluée dans les membranes" [retained in the folds of the womb and adhered to the membranes] (*Caquets* 202).

But, as we know from the scribe's explanation, Guillemeau is not the alleged source of this information. He has learned this from "Madame Perrette, sage-femme du faux-bourg Sainct-Marceau." A midwife is the source of his knowledge. And perhaps not inconsequentially, midwives were often at odds with the male medical establishment in which Guillemeau circulated. In fact, the most famous royal midwife of the period, Louise Boursier, lost her livelihood partially at his son's hands, and over the very issue of an afterbirth allegedly retained in the body of Madame de Montpensier, which was said to have caused her death. In the

Rapport de l'ouverture du corps de feu Madame, Charles Guillemeau and nine other doctors having opened the body, reported the accusatory evidence:

> Au costé droict du fond s'est trouvé une petite portion de l'arriere-faix tellement attachée à la matrice qu'on n'a peu la separer sans peine avec les doigts.
>
> [On the right side at the bottom was found a small portion of the afterbirth so firmly attached to the uterus that one could barely separate it with one's fingers.][29]

Boursier categorically denies this as the cause of death in her lengthy *Fidelle relation de l'accouchement* wherein she meets their accusations head to head, citing many of the ancient and contemporary medical sources to which they also lay claim.[30] She has done her homework, and perhaps relied as well on the wisdom of her husband, who has studied with Ambroise Paré and made available firsthand the knowledge that can exculpate her. The response of the doctors is sour, scornful, and poignantly aligned with this chapter's focus on the birthing body, text, and survival. In the *Remonstrance à Madame Bourcier*, they snarl:

> [V]ous auriez plustost passé tout le reste de vostre vie sans parler, que d'advoüer comme vous faictes (en pensant accuser les Medecins d'inadvertance) que ceste grande Princesse n'a pas esté si bien secourue comme elle le debvoit estre … Les malheurs qui vous sont arrivez trop souvent en l'exercice de vostre vacation et mesme ce dernier qui est du tout deplorable tesmoignent assez vostre suffisance, sans que vous preniez la peine de l'escrire; contentez-vous de nous l'avoir demonstrée à nostre grand dommage, et ne la publiez pas aux Provinces estrangeres … Prevoyez ce qu'on peut tirer de vostre presomption et de vos escris, et ne parlez plus si superbement contre les hommes qui sont plus experimentez et plus heureux que vous en la profession que vous faites. (Rouget and Winn 111–12)

---

[29] This autopsy report is appended in Rouget and Winn's edition of Boursier's writings. Louise Boursier, *Récit véritable de la naissance des messeigneurs et dames les enfans de France; Instruction à ma fille et autres textes*, ed. François Rouget and Colette Winn (Geneva, 2000), p. 109.

[30] As an example, Boursier fires back: "Jamais il ne s'est veu ny leu dans aucun bon Autheur qu'une petite portion de l'arriere-faix deseichée collée contre la matrice sans pourriture eut causé la mort. J'ay leu dans Paul Aeginete en sa Chirurgie que le Medecin ne doit pas s'estonner si une femme n'a vuidé son arriere-faix …" [Never according to any reputable author has it ever been seen or read that a dried up small portion of the afterbirth stuck to the uterus without any rottenness would have caused death. I read in Paul Aeginete in his Surgery that the doctor should not be surprised if a woman has not evacuated her afterbirth] (Rouget and Winn, p. 107).

> [You could have rather spent the rest of your life without speaking rather than admit as you have (wishing to accuse the doctors of wrongdoing) that this great princess had not been as well treated as she should have been … The trials that afflict you all too often in your calling and most surely in this last most deplorable incident are witness enough to your worth, without your having taken the pains to write it; be satisfied at having shown it to us to our great regret and do not publish it in foreign lands … Try and imagine what would be said of the presumption of your writing, and cease from speaking with such superiority against these men who are more experienced and better than you in your profession.]

The afterbirth, then, is attached to womb, to woman, and to gender in a way that makes of this literary trope a singularly political organ: it nourishes, connects, and sustains life just as it has the potential to take it away. It is the prenatal child's bed, the mother's burden, and her delivery, according to the elder Guillemeau, and the accusatory evidence of a woman's incompetence to his son. In fact, for Boursier, the false accusations by these prominent doctors of the period effectively ended her career—a death of another sort. And what is this spate of published defenses and rebuttals if not the afterbirth of a tragic birth event, texts that adhere to the reputations of the interested parties and deliver them (or not) from infamy? The exhortations of Charles Guillemeau and his surgeon friends for Boursier to keep silent, resist publication, and quash her self-defense are desperate and telling. Deliverance indeed. And how additionally ironic that the child born to this mother who died at her lying-in was to become none other than Mademoiselle de Montpensier, a woman of great power, prestige, and prodigious publication!

With this reality in mind, I suggest that the playful, parodic stylings of the erstwhile scribe turned amateur midwife and postpartum mother in the sixth *caquet* are significant in their reach into the valence of the birthing body in early modern lyings-in. The narrator's presumption of women's reproductive capacity is, despite the broad humor evinced throughout the *Recueil*, rich and complex. Certainly, given the references, both direct and implied, to the carnivalesque world of Rabelais, there is reason to interpret this afterbirthed text as derisive, misogynistic, and laughable—all the more to ally it with the critique of the salon/*ruelle* that I have just proposed. And yet I would hold out for a view of this complicated text that might countervail an entirely hopeless, matricidal event, as it were. I would point to the scribe's invocation of Madame Perette, a midwife whose authority is neither derided nor called into question: anti-midwife screeds abound at this time, some so hyperbolic as to fit quite nicely into the more satirical tone of other portions of *Les Caquets*, but this trope is not employed here.[31] Neither the visit of the doctor to

[31] The sixteenth and seventeenth centuries produced a plethora of texts condemning the perpetual incompetency of midwives in favor of male, medical authority. The title alone of Gervais de la Tousche's manual from later in the seventeenth century encapsulates this anxiety quite succinctly: *La Tres-haute et Tres-souveraine science de l'art et industrie*

his postpartum cousin nor the authority of Madame Perette is satirized. Male and female wisdom coexist in much the same way as the cousins share their control and commentary of the spying at the lying-in. The slippage from male to female in the text and the strong female voice of Mathurine and the bathing women from day six suggest this shared authority as well: my pointing to a salon-inspired cast to this collection clearly privileges a more capacious view to gender and authority in this *ruelle*-inspired discourse. And while Domna Stanton's admonishment to call out the misogyny of both this text and its Bakhtinian interpretations is utterly important and convincing, I have brought Gianna Pomata's reconceptualization of the woman's generative body as an alternative way of recuperating this literary event. Her suggestion that the menstruating body was a potentially salutary model of human health and well-being counters an entirely negative view of this comic conceit: bleeding, birthing, and afterbirthing, while all implicated in the rich terrain of the lower stratum so essential to this parody, also implicate the female body in generation and production—both human and literary—that may, wittingly or unwittingly, triumph over its messiness and degradation. In the end, the narrator/scribe does not ridicule his cousin and her generative capacities; he collaborates, and his "afterbirth" is published to great popular acclaim. And so does Louise Boursier, the wrongly accused midwife, make of her afterbirth story a text, a defense against the surgeons who would have her thrown out of any future birthing rooms. Evidence shows that they may have succeeded in practice; but in print, she lives on. Now published along with her *Instruction à ma fille*, a manual that promises the perpetuation of her legacy of sound midwifery to her very own progeny, her "afterbirth," as it were, to this day, validates a woman's right to control her creative and procreative destiny.

naturelle d'enfanster. Contre La Maudicte et Perverse Impericie des femmes que l'on appelle saiges femmes, ou belles meres, lesquelles par leur ignorance font journellement perir une infinité de femmes d'enfans à l'enfantement [The most esteemed and sovereign study of the art and natural industry of childbirthing. Against the malicious and perverse presumption of those women whom we call midwives, or "belles meres," who, by their ignorance cause to perish each day vast numbers of women in childbirth] (Paris, 1587).

Chapter 2
Staging the Competent Midwife: The Royal Birth Stories of François Rabelais and Louise Boursier

> Par cest inconvenient furent au dessus relaschez les cotyledons de la matrice, par lesquelz sursaulta l'enfant, et entra en la vene creuse, et gravant par le diaphragme jusques au dessus des espaules (où ladicte vene se part en deux) print son chemin à gauche, et sortit par l'aureille senestre.
>
> [By this mishap were loosened the cotyledons of the matrix, through which the infant sprang up into the vena cava; and, climbing up by the diaphragm up above the shoulders, where the said vein divides in two, took the route to the left, and came out through the left ear.][1]

Thus culminates one of the most fantastically comical, irreverent, and convoluted birthing stories of all literature: Gargantua's entrance into the world following a labor set in motion by extreme gluttony, vexed by spousal bickering and medical incompetence, and terminated in the most unlikely fashion. As the thirsty giant issues from his startled mother's ear, the reader might well wish to pause, as we shall here, to consider what might be at play in this "accouchement à l'envers": a tale of gargantuan origins at its most crucial, exhilarating, and interpretively charged moments.

In his close reading of Panurge and the Parisian lady in Rabelais's *Pantagruel*—the prequel to *Gargantua*—François Rigolot speaks of such moments as a complex nexus of misogynistic, evangelical, and more contemporary critical discourses. He states:

> Reconstructing a Christian humanist horizon of expectations is an essential step in the hermeneutical process. Just as modern readers must be acquainted with philology to understand the meaning of Rabelais's words, they must also be able to recognize biblical intertexts to grasp the meaning of Rabelais's complex staging of Panurge's misogyny.[2]

---

[1] François Rabelais, *Oeuvres complètes*, ed. Mireille Huchon (Paris, 1994), pp. 21–2. Translation: *The Complete Works of François Rabelais*, Donald M. Frame (Berkeley, 1991), p. 20. All references to Rabelais are from this edition, with translations from Frame's edition. Page numbers are indicated between parentheses in the text.

[2] François Rigolot, "Rabelais, Misogyny, and Christian Charity: Biblical Intertextuality and the Renaissance Crisis of Exemplarity," *PMLA*, 109/2 (1994): p. 233.

The birth of Gargantua is such a "staging" of misogyny. Herein we find a similar confluence of intertexts that, once brought to the discussion, may comment upon the larger debates of women's participation in the telling of and attending to birth taking place in the early modern period. My primary goal here is not to revisit and judge Rabelais's reputation as a misogynist *per se*, but to analyze the discourse he engages in light of other, lesser-known voices operating "in the wings," as it were, of this famous drama.

After reviewing the dramatic event in question and the references that are in play, I put the Rabelaisian text in dialogue with that of another important birth chronicler of the period: the midwife Louise Bourgeois, *dite* Boursier, and specifically her account of the first birth for Marie de Médicis in September, 1601, as related in her *Récit véritable de la naissance de messeigneurs et dames les enfans de France* [*True accounts of the births of the royal children of France*] of 1617. Both Rabelais and Boursier were medical practitioners of their time whose training in the care and maintenance of the human body sharply informed their literary production. While the audiences they address are decidedly different, the ends to which they employ their medical acumen are certainly similar: the legitimizing—either for the sake of heightened comic effect (in the case of Rabelais) or professional reputation (in the case of Boursier)—of the author's medical authority. This chapter indulges a comparison suggested by scholars François Rouget and Colette Winn, who cite at length the birth story of Gargantua in the very first paragraph of the introduction to their superb edition of Boursier's works.[3] Rouget and Winn present the story as participating in a veritable literary industry that decries "l'incompétence des sages-femmes" [the incompetence of midwives] (12). While there is little evidence for a direct textual link between the works of Rabelais and Boursier—Boursier does not refer to Rabelais's *oeuvre* directly at any point—there is a clear and enticing response in her work to the trials endured by midwives so constantly parodied and maligned in print. Boursier counters the prevailing misogyny of the Rabelaisian *cronicques* with her own birth chronicles, which, paired with her more practical gynecological tracts, speak of a mission to legitimize the perennially derided profession to which she lays claim. As Rouget and Winn explain, "[I]l s'agit toujours de transmettre un savoir à la postérité—les couches de la Reine sont des 'cas' aussi intéressants et utiles que ceux répertoriés dans les *Observations*—et de renforcer le prestige et l'autorité de la sage-femme" [Her work is always about the transmission of knowledge for posterity—the Queen's births are "case studies" that are as interesting and useful as those contained in her *Observations*—and about reinforcing the prestige and authority of the midwife] (23).

---

[3] Louise Boursier, *Récit véritable de la naissance de messeigneurs et dames les enfans de France*, ed. François Rouget, and *Instruction à ma fille et autres textes*, ed. Colette Winn (Geneva, 2000). The texts, edited separately, are contained within the same volume; the introductory matter is co-authored. All subsequent references to Boursier's works are from this edition. All translations ae my own unless otherwise noted.

Cathy Hampton's work on what she calls the exemplarity of the case studies, or "body stories," is similarly concerned with gynecological politics and the importance of gender as evidenced in Boursier's work. Her exploration of Boursier's "micro-récit" privileges this midwife as a "textual spokesperson for and translator of the female body in its social as well as medical dimension." She argues:

> In problematizing the relationship between herself and a number of others—women in labour, doctors, her readers—she perceives the necessity to merge skills required in the quasi-scientific endeavours to relieve symptoms with those that anticipate and treat the frailties born of the competing human interests present in the delivery room.[4]

My goal here is to validate this crucial, life-saving (gyn-ecological) mission by comparing Boursier's literary choices with those of Rabelais and with the classical influences that informed them both. Both Rabelais and Boursier are translators of both women's bodies and bodies of writing that they call into service for their dual mission. To be sure, Rabelais's tale transmits a certain strain of knowledge regarding midwives that Boursier's lesser-known example counters with passion and great perspicacity. As in Chapter 1, this comparative reading of Rabelais and Boursier indulges the specter of men in labor and cackling women in a way that ultimately witnesses a woman's recuperation of the birthing body: we are far from the anonymity of *Les Caquets de l'accouchée* as Boursier proudly names herself, her mission, and her destiny.

Gargantuan Birth Stories

Gargantua's birth as retold in the eponymous text is, first, a significant embellishment of its text of origin, the *Grandes cronicques*, which, by comparison, dispenses with the event in rather perfunctory manner. Grandgousier and Gargamelle go off hunting to forget their troubles. The expectant father gallops on ahead after a large herd of deer, slays a dozen of them, and then turns around to see that his wife has not kept up: "Adonc chargea les douze bestes à son col pour veoir où elle estoit demourée. Quant il fut près d'elle, il advisa que elle estoit accouchée et apparçeaut que c'estoit d'ung filz masle" [He then loaded the twelve beasts on his back to go see where she'd gone off to. When he came upon her, he learned that she had already given birth and saw that it was a male child].[5] Grandgousier's feat echoes the third labor of Hercules, the capture of the Hind of Ceryneia. Hercules

[4] Cathy Hampton, "Unpicking Female Exemplarity; or, The Usefulness of Body Stories: Reassessing Female Communal Identity in Two Early Modern French Texts," *Modern Language Review*, 102 (2007): p. 384.

[5] Cited in Roland Antonioli, *Rabelais et la médecine* (Geneva, 1976), p. 165, n. 45.

tracks the illusive deer for a year before throwing it over his neck and returning to appease Eurystheus. Here, then, the *cronicques* project the labor of childbirth onto the *father*, whose Herculean strength, endurance, and exhaustion stand in for the labor and delivery that Gargamelle has been experiencing in his absence, *her* labor cleverly occluded by his.

In the context of Rabelais's *oeuvre*, one also remembers the birth of Gargantua's son, retold in *Pantagruel*. Rabelais's first dramatization of labor-and-delivery stories is significant for what is to be gleaned about midwives and fathers at royal births. In this "prequel" to *Gargantua*, the conditions are tragic: Pantagruel is born healthy but Badebec, his mother, "la fille du Roy des Amaurotes en Utopie," does not survive: "[elle] mourut du mal d'enfant, car il estoit si merveilleusement grand et si lourd, qu'il ne peut venir à lumiere, sans ainsi suffocquer sa mere" [(She) died in childbirth; for he was so wonderfully big and heavy that he could not come into the light of day without choking his mother] (Huchon 222). The attending midwives appear as nothing more competent than gossiping bystanders. To be fair, there is much to astonish: preceding the birth of her child, the attendants look on as a veritable gravy train issues from Badebec's womb: a total of 84 various and sundry beasts of burden, loaded with provisions and pulling along another 25 cartfulls—"ce que espoventa bien lesdictes saiges femmes, mais les aulcunes d'entre elles disoyent. 'Voicy bonne provision aussy bien ne beuyons nous que lachement non en lancement, cecy n'est que bon signe, ce sont aguillons de vin'" [which really terrified the said midwives; but some of them said: "Here are good provisions.You see, we were drinking only meagerly; this is simply a good sign, these are goads to wine"]. The narration continues,

> Et comme elles caquetoyent de ces menus propos entre elles, voicy sorty Pantagruel, tout velu comme un Ours, dont dict une d'elles en esperit propheticque. "Il est né à tout le poil, il fera choses merveilleuses, et s'il vit il aura de l'eage" (224)
>
> [And as they were prattling with one another with such small talk, here comes Pantagruel, all hairy as a bear, and at this in a spirit of prophecy one of them said, "He's born with all his hair on, he'll do wonders; and if he lives, he'll be a grownup"] (Frame 142)

In the context of the tale, this manna arrives to nourish a population in the midst of a terrible drought: the breaking of Badebec's waters, as it were, pours into the midst of a parched world—*tout* ("Panta") *altéré* ("Gruel")—as the author explains in his lengthy meteorological discourse.[6]

[6] See here Edwin Duval's well-known study of Rabelais's structuring of *Pantagruel* within a frame of biblical references, in this moment a response to the Sibylline prophecies of the advent of Christ. Edwin Duval, *The Design of Rabelais's* Pantagruel (New Haven, 1991), p. 17.

Torn between the joy of his son's birth and grief over his wife's passing, Gargantua remains at home writing epitaphs for the deceased Badebec and sends the midwives along to the burial:

> Mais voicy que vous ferez, dict il es saiges femmes (où sont elles bonnes gens, je ne vous peulx veoyr): allez à l'enterrement d'elle, et ce pendent je berceray icy mon filz, car je me sens bien fort alteré, et serois en danger de tomber malade (226)
>
> ["But here's what you do," he said to the midwives. (Where are they? Good folks, I can't see you). "Go to her burial. I'll rock my baby son right here, for I feel quite parched, and might be in danger of falling ill."] (Frame 144)

Here again, the *father* mimics the throes of labor, in this case the pain and grief of his wife's passing, mirroring the exhaustion of the postpartum mother, as Gargantua rocks the newborn Pantagruel to sleep in this *monde a l'envers* that he has just inherited. And the narrator's indictment of the midwives, his irksome plea—"où sont elles bonnes gens, je ne vous peulx veoyr" ["Where are they? Good folks, I can't see you."]—implicitly questions the "sage" in "sages femmes," making the tragedy only that much more lamentable: had they been more "sage" and less *caquette* [gossipy], would things have evolved differently? Rabelais begs the question, and nothing in Gargantua's own birth story to which we turn now is very reassuring.

Gargamelle, resting on the grass after an inadvisably copious feast of tripe and wine, feels the first pangs of labor. Grandgousier responds solicitously, assuring her that the labor will be painful perhaps, but bearable surely, given the joyous miracle that is to ensue. Unconvinced, Gargamelle is reminded of how she got this way and considers aloud the prospects of castration. Exit Grandgousier. Enter the women who are called to oversee this birth:

> Peu de temps aprés elle commença à souspirer, lamenter et crier. Soubdain vindrent à tas saiges femmes de tous coustez. Et la tastant par le bas, trouverent quelques pellauderies, assez de maulvais goust, et pensoient que ce feust l'enfant, mais c'estoit le fondement qui luy escappoit, à la mollification du droict intestine, lequel vous appellez le boyau cullier, par trop avoir mangé des tripes comme avons declairé cy dessus.
>
> Dont une horde vieille de la compaignie, laquelle avoit reputation d'estre grande medicine et là estoit venue de Brizepaille d'auprés Sainct Genou devant soixante ans, luy feist un restrinctif si horrible, que tous ses larrys tant feurent oppilez et reserrez, que à grande poine avesques les dentz, vous les eussiez eslargiz, qui est chose bien horrible à penser. Mesmement que le diable à la messe de sainct Martin escripvant le quaquet de deux gualoises, à belles dentz alongea son parchemin. (21–2)

[A little while after this she began to sigh, lament, and cry out. Immediately there came up midwives in piles from all directions, and, feeling her from below, they found a few lumps of filthy matter with a rather bad taste, and they thought it was the child; but it was the fundament escaping her, from the loosening of the right intestine (which you call the bumgut) from having eaten too many tripes, as we have declared herein above.

Whereas a dirty old hag in the group who had a reputation as a great medic and had come here from Brizepaille near Saint-Genou sixty years before, made her a restringent so horrible that all her sphincters were contracted and tightened up to such a point that you could hardly have pried them open with your teeth; which is a mighty horrible thing to think; in the same way that the devil, writing down the yackety-yack of two old French wenches at Saint Martin's Mass, stretched the parchment just with his teeth.] (Frame 20)

The birth culminates as described in the opening citation. The fantastical nature of Gargantua's birth is heightened in its comic and dramatic effect by the spectacular display of medical detail that Doctor Rabelais packs into his narrative: this is a narrator intimately familiar with medical literature and practice of his time.[7] The comic tension that is established by juxtaposing Rabelais's practical gynecological knowledge with the absurdity of this aural birth is further played out in the misogynistic trope of the incompetent midwives, established as we saw earlier in *Pantagruel*.[8] These women arrive "à tas" [in piles] and "de tous coustez" [from all directions]; the image of their intervention is one of chaos and panic; and their touch, rather than soothing Gargamelle's pain, redoubles it. After they fumble around "par le bas," they are quick to misdiagnose: a competent assistant might have read about such "pellauderies" or prolapses of the intestinal wall or vagina and certainly not mistaken them for the child, or been so bungling in the execution of what was actually a standard remedy.[9] Rabelais immediately corrects their

7 I recall here my earlier conjecture that the narrator of *Les Caquets de l'accouchée* was similarly enamored with medical knowledge and may well have been trained in medicine himself (see Chapter 1). For a treatment of the classical allusions to monstrous or fantastical births, see Jean-Marie Jacques, "Sur l'accouchement de Gargamelle," *Bulletin de l'Association des amis de Rabelais et de La Devinière*, 4/10 (1991): pp. 396–400; Antonioli, *Rabelais et la médecine*, remains quite useful in its analysis of contemporaneous medical discourse as alluded to in the work of Rabelais.

8 Others have remarked upon the poignant connections here between the Christian and Gargantuan nativities. If Christ was *conceived* through Mary's ear at the annunciation, Gargantua brings this exquisitely cerebral and spiritual allusion to its most literally mind-numbing conclusion: Gargantua, who comes to reign and revel in the issue of all appetites, is *born* from the ear as well. See Michaël Baraz, *Rabelais et la joie de la liberté* (Paris, 1983), p. 236, and Antonioli, *Rabelais et la médecine*, p. 170.

9 A counter-scenario for the birth attendant's intervention at this crucial stage of delivery can be found in Jacques Guillemeau's *De l'Heureux accouchement des femmes...*,

diagnosis with his firm command of the situation: "*mais* c'estoit le fondement qui luy escappoit, à la mollification du droict intestine, lequel *vous appellez* le boyau cullier …" [*but* it was the fundament escaping her, from the loosening of the right intestine, which *you call* the bumgut] (my emphasis). Contrary to their misguided assumptions, Rabelais knows quite precisely what has happened and entreats the reader ("vous") to believe and agree. The narrator invites a designated readership of learned, level-headed practitioners in opposition to the "elles," the meddling midwives or female medical assistants.

Certainly the specter of the "horde vieille," the dirty old hag from Brizepaille, does nothing to inspire confidence in women's competency: "grande medicine" indeed, who would set in motion such a disastrous delivery.[10] Gargantua, thanks to the misguided ministrations of this old hag, is propelled through the laboring body of Gargamelle, traveling along a route that, while seemingly unnavigable, is grounded in received medical knowledge of the day. As Antonioli explicates:

> Mais la matrice est reliée au foie par divers vaisseaux nourriciers qui n'ont pas de nom dans l'anatomie du temps. Elle a, d'autre part, comme le montre Mondino de Luzzi, des connexions veineuses avec la veine cave ascendante … qui ne passent pas par le foie. Enfin Gargantua dispose encore, dans cette partie médiane du voyage, d'un troisième itinéraire possible, par la veine cave descendante dans laquelle viennent s'ouvrir les vaisseaux spermatiques qui débouchent, à leur tour, dans la matrice. (Antonioli 169)

> [But the uterus is connected to the liver by various feeder vessels which had no name in the anatomy of the time. It [the uterus] had, as well, as shown by Mondino de Luzzi, venous connections with the ascending vena cava … which did not pass through the liver. Finally, Gargantua has at his disposal a third

---

which suggests precisely the opposite effect of a well-applied stringent. The surgeon (the "chirurgien" is clearly Guillemeau's preference here) should hasten the birth of a weakening child, encouraging the mother as best as possible, "luy faisant par en bas, & principalement vers le siege & os pubis, qui sont les deux extremitez du conduict naturel, de petits linimens avec le bout & extremité des doigts ... Ce qui fera irriter à esguillonner la matrice à l'expulsion dudit enfant" [administering to her nether regions, and principally to her seat and the pubic bone, which are at the furthest extremity of their natural course, some liniments with the very ends of the fingers … which will irritate and contract the womb in order to expulse the child.] Jacques Guillemeau, *De l'Heureux accouchement des femmes où il est traicté du gouvernement de leur grossesse, de leur travail naturel et contre nature, du traictement estant accouchées et de leurs maladies* (Paris, 1609), p. 217.

[10] According to the Ducat edition of 1711 cited in the Huchon edition, "En languedoc et en Daulphiné, dire d'une femme qu'elle est venue de Brisepaille, d'auprès de Sainct-Genou … c'est désigner une vieille débauchée" [In the Languedoc and Dauphiné regions, to speak of a woman as coming from Brisepaille, near Saint-Genou … is to taint her as a debauched old woman]. Huchon, *Oeuvres complètes*, p. 1080, n. 7.

possible route in this middle portion of his travels, by way of the descending vena cava into which the sperm vessels discharge in turn into the uterus.]

By contrast with these "piles" or "masses" of ignorant midwives, Rabelais establishes a medical discourse that heightens the show of their incompetence while displaying, however humorously, his mastery of medical knowledge.

The send-up of meddling women is complemented finally in Rabelais's allusion to the devil and the Mass of Saint Martin. Gargamelle's incompetent female assistants are smeared only further when compared to the three gossips who, according to the legend, chattered their way through Mass as the devil recorded their every word; so lengthy was their irreverent cackling that the demonic scribe was forced to lengthen his parchment with his teeth, eventually tearing it, stumbling back, falling, and breaking his neck.[11] The carnal terrain here is rich: Rabelais compares the stretched parchment (which would connote at this time vellum or animal hide) and the recording of impertinent gossip to the constricted, vaginal membranes of the birthing giantess, while at the same time leading the reader to imagine *himself*, his head in the lap of Gargamelle, attempting to secure an exit for this monstrous birth—"à grande poine avesques les dentz, *vous* les eussiez eslargiz" [you could hardly have pried them open with your teeth]. We, Rabelais's readers, are now asked to move in ever closer to the unappetizing site of Gargamelle's "pellauderies, assez de maulvais goust" [lumps of filthy matter with a rather bad taste]. In true carnivalesque mode, the upper and lower body are confused and reversed: the birthing child erupts up and out of Gargamelle's head and our (the reader's) head is directed down to the stretched membranes of her reproductive organs. Rabelais asks us to imagine the smells, the tastes, and the feel of Gargamelle's birthing body in the most primal of ways; like the devil at Saint Martin's Mass we chew on this woman/text, this putrid, distasteful, and resistant "parchment" that Rabelais sets before us.

This gendered, medical horizon of expectations presents an array of information to be interrogated: Why the association of midwives and impertinent gossips at this legendary birth? What is at stake in the distinction that Rabelais draws between his fraternal reader—"*vous* appellez le boyau," "*vous* les eussiez eslargiz"—and these ignorant, foolish women? In a society rife with the tension of increasingly

[11] See here Caroline Bicks's references to the conflation of gossips and midwives: "The gossip, the nurse, the midwife and the mother (distinct women to be sure) at times become interchangeable in the texts that portray them, since all four shared in the touches and tales that midwived subjects into being," *Midwiving Subjects in Shakespeare's England* (Aldershot, 2003), p. 12. We have already seen in this chapter the characterization of women, midwifery, and cackling that are so consistently connected in Rabelais: "Et comme elles *caquetoyent* de ces menus propos entre elles" and "sainct Martin escripvant le *quaquet* de deux gualoises" (my emphasis), the misogynistic *Zeitgeist* that nourishes full-blown indulgence in texts such as Chapter 1's *Les Caquets de l'accouchée*.

medicalized childbirth, where is the doctor? Where is the midwife? What is being born, that is to say, (re)produced?

One can respond to "Where's the doctor?" by returning to the incompetent "grande médecine" of Brizepaille and to Rabelais, author and doctor with authority not only over his text, but also over real women's birthing bodies of his day. This birth story is one of disorder, surely, but also of control: while the hordes of incompetent midwives and the quack woman doctor from Brizepaille infuse this scene with utter calamity, the narrative and medical authority belongs to Doctor Rabelais. Absent any competent medical professional, this doctor/author will have to do. He establishes a pact between himself and "vous," a fraternity of readers who laugh along with him at the incompetence of bumbling women. So then, Rabelais asks us through his allusion to the legend of Saint Martin, to imagine the laboring, contracting, constricting woman's body as a text—literally—that he will inscribe. Like the "laboring" and "postpartum" fathers whom Rabelais so comically depicts in his birth stories, his message is most importantly about men and male authority; the women, Gargamelle and her midwives and attendants, are depicted as cantankerous, incompetent, and meddlesome, respectively. Rabelais's men appropriate their labor on both accounts: as fathers suffering from the strain of their wives' physical ordeal and as the true medical authorities who "labor" at the bedside of these crazed mothers-to-be. This comedy of errors, infused as it is with the tropes of women's inadvisable participation in royal births, is a decidedly masculinist version of the pitfalls of parturition. For the feminist version: enter Louise Boursier.

Is There a Midwife in the Château?

To the questions about male and female medical authority I have posed, I propose a reading of Rabelais's text and the misogynistic assumptions it reproduces alongside the example of an actual midwife of the period—a woman, who, like Rabelais, appeared also to enjoy good storytelling with more than a little comic relief. The midwife Louise Boursier (1563–1636), who began practice at the end of the sixteenth century in Paris, was, like Rabelais, a chronicler whose narratives of childbirth were all the more riveting for her experience, and her unassailable competence. Also like Rabelais, the birthing woman's body is her text, her way into writing and self-legitimation.

The juxtaposition of texts I interrogate here participates in a recent burgeoning of scholarship over the last decade that has investigated the disputes between male and female medical practitioners of the period. Wendy Perkins's groundbreaking study of Boursier's writings and career presents the polemics of the debate in historical detail, while modern editions of Boursier's work have spurred further scholarship, most notably with respect to women's agency and control in the early modern period. While these studies do not agree uniformly, most notably on the issue of woman's exclusion and denigration within the male medical establishment, the central question of the control of women's bodies and reproduction—taken within this chapter as both literal and literary—remains provocative and revealing, however, of practices and attitudes that illuminate questions of gender and power at this time.[12]

Louise Boursier was the renowned midwife to many of the Parisian elite, including, on six occasions, Marie de Médicis. She wrote at length of her experiences in several books, including *Observations diverses sur la stérilité, perte de fruits, fécondité, accouchements et maladies des femmes et enfants nouveau-nés suivi de Instruction à ma fille* [*Some observations on sterility, miscarriage, fecundity, births and illnesses of women and newborns, followed by Instructions to my daughter*] of 1609 and the *Récit véritable de la naissance de messeigneurs et dames les enfans de France* [*The true account of the births of the royal children of France*] of 1617. As a midwife with literary pretensions, Boursier is at the nexus of an array of issues concerning the coopting of midwives' livelihood by the university-trained male medical establishment and the persistent suspicion of women's published self-expression.[13] Boursier was, however, in a unique and privileged position within the medical fraternity, as we see in the opening pages of her *Instruction à ma fille* where she reminds her daughter, "un Docteur en medecine est mary de vostre sœur, vostre mary fait son cours pour l'estre, l'un de vos freres est Pharmacien, vostre pere est Chirurgien, et moy sage-femme; le corps de la medecine est entier dans nostre maison." [Your sister's husband is a doctor of medicine, your husband is studying to be one, one of your brothers is a Pharmacist, your father is a Surgeon and I, a midwife; the entire medical establishment exists within your household] (Rouget and Winn 124). Boursier therefore negotiates the prevalent misogyny parodied by Rabelais from within: she is indebted to these learned men for much of her knowledge and speaks from

[12] See Wendy Perkins, *Midwifery and Medicine in Early Modern France: Louise Bourgeois* (Exeter, 1996); Louise Bourgeois, *dite* Boursier, *Observations diverses, sur la sterilité, perte de fruict, accouchements, et maladies des femmes, et enfants nouveaux naiz* (1609), ed. Françoise Olive (Paris, 1992) and *Récit véritable*; Bicks, *Midwiving Subjects*; Lianne McTavish, *Childbirth and the Display of Authority in Early Modern France* (Aldershot, 2005); Susan Broomhall, *Women's Medical Work in Early Modern France* (Manchester, 2004).

[13] On the severity of this rift along gender lines, some scholars part company. Responding sympathetically to the notion of masculinity in crisis rather than control, McTavish proposes that male midwives fared no better than females; while male midwifery is not at issue directly with Boursier, the subject is clearly heating up at the time of the *Récits*, and the gender of birth attendants at any level was crucial to the debate: "I likewise find that early modern French masculinity was insecure, rather than all powerful. Men-midwives emerge from obstetrical treatises as unsteady figures who, like women, were subject to scrutiny in the lying-in chamber," *Childbirth and the Display of Authority*, p. 10. While the newly emerging class of men-midwives proves an interesting gray area in the polemic, I propose that male medical authority of the university-trained level still prevailed to the exclusion of women's voice and experience.

a highly privileged position that most other midwives did not enjoy; despite this privilege, Boursier went on to suffer intense vilification and condemnation by other members of the medical community for perceived incompetence as midwife to Madame de Montpensier, who died in childbirth; the scandal appears to have ended Boursier's career at court—not, however, without a spate of accusations and defenses in print by both sides.[14]

Boursier's publications recount a number of births that she attended. Many of the anecdotes serve as examples of particular difficulties associated with her profession; some, as in the case we now turn to—the birth of the future Louis XIII—serve as both self-promotion and historical record. Just as Gargantua's birth is situated within a context of literary precedents and medical authority that prepare its reception (see Chapter I of *Gargantua*: "De la genealogie et antiquité de Gargantua"), so is Boursier's account of the dauphin's birth allied with a lineage that assures our confidence. As demonstrated just above, Boursier, in her first publication that she dedicates to her daughter, establishes her own family's professional legitimacy: Boursier's daughter is born into the rarefied upper echelon of the Parisian medical establishment. If Boursier's genealogy comprises only several generations (as opposed to the noble, ancient Assyrian beginnings of Gargantua!), her dedication does also connect herself (and her daughter) to a classical sorority: "Me trouvant embarquée dans un ménage, chargée d'enfants, accablée de guerre et de perte de bien, la sage Phanerote, mère de ce grand philosophe Socrate, prit pitié de moi" [Finding myself launched into a household, weighed down by children, beseiged by war and the loss of wealth, the wise Phanerote, mother of the great philosopher Socrates, took pity on me] (124). Boursier invokes an ancestor here from Plato's *Theatetus*, whose point about Socrates's mother was that she, as an attendant to *women's* bodies, was patently less worthy and noble than her son, who helped birth *men's* souls. Boursier is happy to reclaim her, and Lucina as well, the goddess of childbirth, who in Ovidian myth exhibits fantastic and powerful control over women's bodies in labor.[15]

---

[14] See the conclusion of Chapter 1. The record of this was quite public and is chronicled in a series of publications regarding the scandal that effectively ended her career: the *Fidelle relation de l'accouchement, maladie et ourverture du corps de feu Madame* (1627); the *Rapport de l'ouverture du corps de feu Madame* (1627); and the *Remonstrance à Madame Bourcier, touchant son Apologie* (1627) in Rouget and Winn, pp. 97–120. See also Perkins, *Midwifery and Medicine*, p. 25.

[15] Boursier speaks of herself as "estant petite fille de Phanerote, disciple de Lucine, maistresse de Mercure, à cause que Lucine l'a assujetty à vostre mere" [the grand-daughter of Phanerote, disciple of Lucina, mistress of Mercury, the result of which was to enslave her to your mother] (Rouget and Winn, p. 124). On Lucina, see Ovid, *Metamorphoses*, Books IX and X, especially the story of Alcmene's labor. We are reminded here as well of the ways in which the labors of Gargamelle (from the *Cronicques*) and Badebec are appropriated by their husbands as previously observed.

If Gargamelle's delivery unfolds, presumably "sur l'herbe" after her nasty bout of tripe-induced indigestion, Marie de Médicis's 22-hour ordeal is staged, quite literally, in the most grandiose and orderly of fashions:

> [U]n grand lict de velours de cramoisi rouge accommodé d'or, estoit prés le lict de travail, aussi les pavillons, le grand et le petit, qui estoient attachez au plancher, et troussez, furent destroussez. Le grand pavillon fut tendu ainsi qu'une tente par les quatre coins avec cordons; il estoit d'une belle toille de Hollande, et avoit bien vingt aulnes de tour, au milieu duquel il y en avoit un petit de pareille toille, sous lequel fut mis le lict de travail, où la Roine fut couchée au sortir de sa chambre. (Rouget and Winn 75)

> [A large bed of crushed red velvet, trimmed in gold, was next to the labor bed; also the canopies, large and small, which were nailed to the floor and then trussed up, were let down. The large canopy was stretched over like a tent from the four corners with ropes; it was made of a beautiful toile from Holland, 72 feet around, in the middle of which there was another canopy of the same fabric, under which was placed the labor bed where the Queen was placed just outside her bedroom.]

There is nothing in this description to suggest that the production was any less extravagant than the painterly renditions by Rubens in his gigantic canvases of this and other events in the life of Marie de Médicis now housed in the Louvre. If the physical stage is set beautifully, the attention to the movements of the cast of characters is equally deft: Boursier comforts the queen throughout; she attends to the first and second ladies-in-waiting, each jealous of the other over who shall be informed of the sex of the child first. A system of secret signals is created: for the first lady: "la Reine estant accouchée d'un fils, je devois baisser la teste en signe que tout alloit bien; si c'eust esté une fille, je la devois renverser en arriere" [Should the Queen give birth to a son, I was to lower my head as a sign that all was going well; if it was a girl, I was to tip it back] (72); for the second: "que je lui disse tout haut, si tost que la Reine seroit accouchée d'un fils: 'Ma fille, chauffe-moi un linge'" [I was to say to her as soon as the Queen bore a son: "My girl, warm me some linens"] (73). The women then proceed to tell the happy news to the incredulous king. In Boursier's account, the king can only be assured by addressing her directly:

> La couleur revint au Roy, et vint à moy à costé de la Reine, et se baissa, et mit la bouche contre mon oreille, et me demanda: "Sage-femme est-ce un fils?" Je lui dis qu'ouy. "Je vous prie, ne me donnez point de corte-joye, cela me feroit mourir." Je desvelope un petit Monsieur le Dauphin, et lui fis voir que c'estoit un fils, que la Reine n'en vit rien. Il leva les yeux au Ciel aiant les mains jointes, et rendit graces à Dieu. Les larmes lui couloient sur la face, aussi grosses que de gros pois. (79)

> [The King's color came back, and he came to me next to the Queen, bent over, placed his mouth against my ear and asked: "Midwife, is it a son?" I answered "Yes." "I beg of you, don't just say that to make me happy, I would die if this weren't true." I uncovered just a bit Monsieur le Dauphin, and showed him that it was indeed a son, being careful that the Queen saw nothing. He raised his eyes to Heaven, joined his hands, and thanked God. Tears as large as fat peas streamed down his face.]

Boursier's comic tenderness here, the pea-like tears worthy of Rabelais, to be sure, converges in an intimacy with the king—"la bouche contre mon oreille" [his mouth against my ear]—that confers upon her the ultimate authority. She commands these characters in every way.

The frenetic intrigue of the announcement of the infant's sex is also commensurate with a detail from Gargantua's birth, namely, Chapter III, "Comment Gargantua fut unze moys porté ou ventre de sa mere" ["How Gargantua was Carried Eleven Months in His Mother's Belly"]. It is likely, as Antonioli suggests, that Rabelais's first impulse here is to connect Gargantua's birth to a historical, literary tradition: "C'est, en effet, une convention épique, comme le rappelle Rabelais, que les enfants illustres, par leur origine ou par leur destinée, aient une gestation plus longue que la durée normale" [It is, in fact, an epic convention that Rabelais refers to, that famous children, given their origins and destiny, undergo a longer than normal gestation] (Antonioli 161). Antonioli follows, moreover, with a commentary on the legal, moral, and political ramifications of the accuracy of such information: a son was clearly cause for greater celebration, but a son born within the credible time-frame associated with the coupling of his parents was also at issue. Midwives such as Boursier were privy to such knowledge and remanded to be most judicious in their confidences and steadfast if called before interested legal authority. Rabelais the jurist perhaps reminds us of the peculiarities of gestational indeterminacy as he concludes the chapter with accounts of the plight of the recently widowed preyed upon by over-eager suitors: "Car si au troisiesme moys elles engroissent: leur fruict sera heritier du deffunct" [Because if by the third month they are pregnant, their offspring will be the legal inheritor of the deceased] (Huchon 16). Boursier's account is scrupulous in its detailing of the moment of actual birth: "Il estoit dix heures et demie du soir, le Jeudy xxvij. Septembre mil six cens un, jour de Saint-Cosme et Saint-Damian, neuf mois et quatorze jours apres le mariage de la Reine" [It was ten thirty in the evening, Thursday the 27th. September, sixteen hundred and one, feast day of Saint-Cosme and Saint-Damian, nine months and fourteen days after the Queen's marriage] (Rouget and Winn 80). Both Rabelais and Boursier suggest the serious consequences stirring in these tears "as large as fat peas."

Boursier's account of the dauphin's entrance into the world is one of perpetual judicious oversight in the face of an anxiety-ridden court. Her authority is absolutely central to the success of the birth; her narrative is all the more credible and engaging for the way in which she humanizes the drama around her. Just as even the contemporary reader of Rabelais is bemused by the classically misguided and poorly received consolations of Grandgousier to his laboring wife, so does the plight of Boursier and her long-suffering queen not fail to entertain. The king is insistent that the blood princes be present and presses his wife to comply:

> M'amie, vous sçavez que je vous ay dit par plusieurs fois le besoin qu'il y a que les Princes du Sang soient à vostre accouchement. Je vous supplie de vous y vouloir resoudre, c'est la grandeur de vous et de vostre enfant. (73)

> [My love, you know how I've told you several times the necessity of having the blood princes at your delivery. I implore you to resign yourself to this, for the greatness of you and your child.]

At one in the morning the king, "vaincu d'impatience," calls in the princes against better judgment, declaring, playfully:

> Si jamais l'on a veu trois Princes en grand'peine, l'on en verra tantost, ce sont trois Princes grandement pitoiables et de bon naturel, qui voiant souffrir ma femme voudroient pour beaucoup de leur bien estre bien loing d'ici. (74)

> [If we've never seen three Princes in great suffering, we shall see it soon; these are three Princes, much to be pitied and of a kindly disposition, who, upon seeing my wife in agony, will wish they were far from here.]

Not words of great succor, certainly, for his wife who, according to Boursier's account, is still a good 21 hours away from delivering. That she pretends to speak in the voice of the king and report his speech directly is further evidence of her sense of entitlement in the rarefied atmosphere of the dauphin's birth chamber.

The royal youth remain continuously underfoot throughout the delivery. Boursier's anecdote regarding the petulant young Duc de Vendôme is telling for its relevance regarding this particular midwife's sense of privilege and authority. She describes the duke's query:

> Il me demandoit à toute heure si la Reine accoucheroit bientost, et de quel enfant ce seroit. Pour le contenter, je lui dis qu'oui. Il me demanda derechef quel enfant ce seroit; je lui dis que ce seroit ce que je voudrois. "Et quoi, dit-il, n'est-il pas fait?" Je lui dis qu'ouy, qu'il estoit enfant, mais que j'en ferois un fils ou une fille, ainsi qu'il me plairoit. Il me dit: "Sage-femme, puisque cela dépend de vous, mettez y les pieces d'un fils!" (77)

> [He was constantly asking me if the Queen would deliver soon and what kind of child it would be. To appease him, I said "yes." He then asked immediately what kind; I told him it would be what I wanted. "What?" he said, "Is it not already done?" I responded that yes, it was already a child, but that I would make of it a

> boy or a girl, as I pleased. He said to me: "Midwife, since it all depends on you, put on the boy's parts!"]

Boursier's response is a playful retort to this naive youth, but a more pointed self-promotion for her readers: her will be done "ce que je voudrois," "ainsi qu'il me plairoit." The interchange gives her an opportunity to name herself ("Sage-femme") and legitimize herself ("puisque cela dépend de vous")—albeit in a whimsical and humorous fashion. Her good humor is, indeed, her hallmark, as the royal spectacle began with practical jokes—"J'estois couchée dans la garde-robbe de la Reine, où souvent pour rire on me donnoit de fausses allarmes" [I was asleep in the Queen's wardrobe, where for a laugh, they kept waking me up with false alarms] (73)—and terminates with the storming of the bedchamber by literally hundreds of desperate well-wishers who clearly try her patience: "Je croy qu'il y avoit deux cens personnes, de sorte que l'on ne pouvoit se remuer dans la chambre pour porter la Reine dans son lict" [I believe there were 200 people, so many that one couldn't even turn around in the room to carry the Queen to her bed] (80). In the end, recognizing the sex of the newborn is the drama's stirring climax. Boursier moves between the queen's legs for the final moments of delivery, and reserves for herself alone the first sight. She will be the first to know, the first to tell. That she pretends to have a hand (literally) in determining the sex of the much yearned-for male heir is at once humorous and suggestive of her all-encompassing supremacy in this affair.

Finally, a close reading of this climactic scene reveals once again the ways in which Boursier consciously responds to the misogynistic strains within the medical hierarchy, culminating in a dénouement that gestures at once critically and sympathetically to the Rabelaisian text. If Gargamelle's labor onset was at first mistaken for indigestion, Boursier would have been familiar with the pregnant woman's dietary peculiarities and assessed the situation more masterfully. In the *Observations diverses*, she speaks of detecting pregnancy:

> Il faut savoir si elles ont perdu l'appétit des viandes que de tout temps elles avaient accoutumé d'aimer. Si elles ont eu envie de viandes nouvelles … il leur semble que tout ce qui leur touche au corps les blesse, et spécialement après avoir mangé pour peu que ce soit.[16]
>
> [One must know if they have lost their appetite for foods they previously enjoyed. If they have had new cravings … if it seems that anything that touches them irritates, and especially after having eaten however small a quantity.]

During the queen's labor, she performs her duties in this regard, again with typical aplomb, this time evincing her medical superiority in no uncertain terms:

---

16 Boursier, *Observations*, p. 57.

> Sur les quatre heures du matin, une grande colique se mesla parmi le travail de la Reine, qui lui donna d'extremes douleurs, sans avancement. De fois à autre le Roi faisoit venir les Medecins veoir la Reine, et me parler, ausquels je rendois compte de ce qui se passoit … Les Medecins me demanderent: "Si c'estoit une femme où n'y eust que vous pour la gouverner, que lui feriez-vous?" Je leur proposay des remedes qu'ils ordonnerent à l'instant à l'Apoticaire. (76)

> [Around four in the morning, the Queen's labor was interrupted by great indigestion which gave her severe contractions with no advancement in labor. From time to time the King called in the Doctors to see the Queen, and to speak with me, at which time I gave them an update … The Doctors asked me: "If this were a woman who had only you to look after her, what would you do?" I proposed several remedies that they ordered immediately from the Apothecary.]

The calling in of male doctors at any labor was being done with increasing frequency, and Boursier illustrates here the tensions in play between the traditional midwife's longstanding practical knowledge and experience and the male doctor's reliance on the book. Boursier embodies both: she has attended hundreds of births by now and clearly had a stockpile of remedies that she published during her years as royal midwife.[17] She reproduces here the conversation that betrays the male medical authority's reliance on her which allows her to display her successful response. This resolution of the queen's secondary discomfort has resonance in ways that hint at an empowering of women's voice within the delivery room that is poignant and dramatic.

> Lorsque les remedes eurent dissipé la colique et que la Reine alloit accoucher, je voiois qu'elle se retenoit de crier; je la suppliay de ne s'en retenir de peur que sa gorge ne s'enflât. Le roi lui dit: "M'amie, faites ce que vostre sage-femme vous dit, criez de peur que vostre gorge s'enfle." (78)

> [When the remedies had dissipated the indigestion and the Queen was about to give birth, I noticed that she was restraining herself from crying out; I implored here not to hold back for fear that her throat swell up. The king said: "My love, do as your midwife tells you, cry out so that your throat doesn't swell up."]

Boursier's remedy has released the queen from digestive discomfort and now it remains to push her labor to its final stage. Once again, Boursier presents the scene in such as way as to report the king's actual speech, advice that admonishes his wife to trust in Boursier, cry out, and release herself from this interminable labor.

---

[17] Boursier's *Observations diverses* includes a great number of remedies for various stages of labor, concluding, in fact, with "Remède pour apaiser le vomissement." *Observations*, p. 220.

Throughout the lengthy account of the dauphin's birth, the queen has remained entirely mute—in great contrast with the constant interjections of the myriad attendants milling about the room, from toddling princes and dukes to nervous doctors to the panicky royal patriarch. Here, Boursier releases her from this silence and her cry sets in motion the happy miracle that assures the monarchy its future. If Gargamelle's bizarre, inverted labor is propelled by the intensity of corporeal restriction occasioned by the incompetent medical "hag," Marie de Médicis's agony is resolved by unconstricting, opening up, giving voice to both her and her midwife—"faites ce que vostre sage-femme vous dit"—an act of maternal initiation and of self-legitimation for the queen and the midwife respectively.

The final dénouement is equally inspired and well staged. The crying out is successful; the queen is brought to the birthing chair and Boursier moves in between her legs to receive the baby. Boursier has exclusive control over the crucial last moment:

> J'estois sur un petit siege devant la Reine, laquelle estant accouchée, je mis Monsieur le Dauphin dans des linges et langes dans mon giron sans que personne sceut que moi quel enfant c'estoit. Je l'enveloppai bien, ainsi que j'entendois à ce que j'avois affaire. (78)
>
> [I was on a small seat before the Queen who had just given birth and I swaddled Monsieur le Dauphin and put him close to my chest so that no one but I would know what kind of child it was. I wrapped him up well following what I knew I should do.]

The dauphin is weak from so much time in the birth canal and Boursier ruminates aloud about possible remedies, leery of following her instincts, given the clientele: her *Observations diverses* make it clear that the practice of giving a small quantity of wine to the newborn to give it a start would be her preferred way to proceed.[18] She addresses the king:

> "SIRE, si c'estoit un autre enfant je mettrois du vin dans la bouche, et lui en donnerois, de peur que la foiblesse dure trop." Le Roy me mit la bouteille contre la bouche et me dit: "Faites comme à un autre." J'emplis ma bouche de vin et lui en soufflay; à l'heure mesme il revint, et savoura le vin que je lui avois donné. (78)

[18] This is advice garnered from "learned doctors" (perhaps those of her own family) that Boursier has trusted and here cites as helpful. From the chapter "De ce qui se doit faire aux enfants sitôt qu'ils sont nés": "J'ai vu tenir pour maxime à des médecins fort doctes que sitôt qu'un enfant est né, il lui faut donner à prendre une petite cuillerée de vin pur, disant qu'il aide l'enfant à reprendre ses esprits ..." *Observations*, p. 95.

> ["My Lord, if this were any other child, I would place a little wine in my mouth and give him a little for fear that his weak state last too long." The King placed the bottle against my mouth and said: "Do as you would with any other." I filled my mouth with wine and blew out a bit into the baby's; he came to right away and savored the wine that I had just given him.]

The scene presents, once again, a spectacle of intense physical intimacy: Boursier's hands in the queen's lap and on the dauphin as he issues from the womb; the king placing the bottle of wine against her mouth; and finally, Boursier, her lips against those of the newborn child, literally inspiring him with a revitalizing drink. There is a convergence of maternal, erotic, and religious communion in the intimacy of these final moments that is arresting and all but hagiographic in the power and centrality it bestows upon Boursier. As commanding and supremely trustworthy midwife to the queen, as confidante to the king in his most vulnerable entrance into fatherhood, and as the first to hold the dauphin to her breast, Boursier stars in a production of spectacular self-promotion.

"A boire! A boire!" [Some drink! Some drink!], cries the newborn Gargantua in his first earthly utterance. The dauphin, too, savors his way into the world, yet in his case in the arms of a most unassailably competent female medical authority. There is much to savor and rejoice in at this birth, not the least of which is the successful (re)production of women's voice and control—a narrative steeped in drama, gynecological erudition, and more than a little good humor. Boursier grants us another chronicle of royal childbirth that gives Rabelais and his Gargantua their due.

***

As stated at the outset, there was never an *actual* dialogue between Rabelais and Boursier (though the prospect of such an encounter would make for a feisty *dialogue des morts*, no doubt). The juxtaposition of their discourses, however, illuminates a struggle fueled by misogynist banter of no small consequence. Rabelais's allusion to the devil's recording of the gossips at Saint Martin's bespeaks a risible sorority of miscreants, whose "caquettage" is so longwinded that it stretches (literally) the limits of the devil's notebook—a characterization made all the more unseemly by its association with the straining genitals of Gargamelle. Boursier takes up her own notebook and offers us another lengthy narrative, but in utter opposition to the trivialities of the gossips of Saint Martin's or Rabelais's chattering, nattering midwives. Her story is at once controlled, humorous, instructive, and, in the context of such parodies as that of Rabelais, redemptive. The dénouement is set in motion by the queen's crying out, an act suggested and permitted by Boursier and redolent of the courage and competence of her own project of empowerment. To revisit our earlier queries: Where is the doctor? Following orders. Where is the midwife? Center stage. What is being born (reproduced)? The next French monarch, to be sure; but also a version of the proceedings that tells of women's strength and engagement in a noble profession. As Boursier philosophizes in her final words to her daughter in the *Instruction*:

> … depuis que le monde est, il y a tousjours eu un grand discord entre la verité et le mensonge, mais quelques subtilitez que le mensonge aye peu aporter contre la verité, elle est demeurée victorieuse. (Rouget and Winn 144)
>
> [… from the beginning of time, there has always been a struggle between truth and lies, but despite the small, subtle gains of lies against truth, truth always triumphs.]

Boursier's work speaks truth to the power of her day. As her queen cries out, so does she in this eloquent testimony to rival even the most gargantuan of tales.

Chapter 3
Touching and Telling: Gendered Variations on a Gynecological Theme

Childbirth for women at the turn of the sixteenth century was at once life-giving and life-threatening; to bring children into the world was to put oneself in danger. Birthing children of the mind through writing and publishing was an equally perilous enterprise for women in a society that marked all of their reproductive capacities, both biological and intellectual, with shame and suspicion. An investigation of the writings of both men and women surrounding childbirth can prove fruitful regarding the limits and possibilities of women's expression, both of the body and the spirit.

The perception of childbirth as a dangerous event in the life of early modern women is the subject of no little debate, and the language and arguments used for framing the polemic are instructive in and of themselves. Lianne McTavish is wont to question overly dire statistics. She sees the exaggeration of reports on maternal mortality as participating in a transhistorical misogynistic tradition of condemning midwives' incompetency. She says of recent historians of medicine, "By undertaking careful archival research, they have undermined longstanding assumptions about early modern childbirth. It is no longer possible to presume that female midwives were incompetent, women had no control over conception, and birth itself was extremely dangerous."[1] McTavish responds to the conventional and repeated wisdom of scholars such as Lawrence Stone, who generalize broadly from what seems like much of the cautionary, hyperbolic literature from the early modern period: "For women, childbirth was a very dangerous experience, for midwives were ignorant and ill trained, and often horribly botched the job, while the lack of hygienic precautions meant that puerperal fever was a frequent sequel."[2] Commensurate with such predictions is the speculation of B.M. Willmott Dobbie, whose prose betrays not only the general mystery of the birthing process in the early modern era, but also our knowledge of its history from that time to the present:

---

1 Lianne McTavish, *Childbirth and the Display of Authority in Early Modern France* (Aldershot, 2005), p. 8.

2 Lawrence Stone, *The Family, Sex, and Marriage in England 1500–1800* (New York, 1977), p. 79. For countervailing argument and evidence in a variety of European examples, see Roger Schofield's "Did the Mothers Really Die? Three Centuries of Maternal Mortality in 'The World We Have Lost'," in *The World We Have Gained: Histories of Population and Social Structure* (New York, 1986).

> An enquiry into family structure in previous centuries reveals evidence of the high price in women's lives of replenishment of the population. It could not be otherwise, for when Nature failed in her task, or was thwarted by such adversities as pelvic deformity or malpresentation, attempts to help were mostly fumbling in the dark, literally and metaphorically, and well-meant interference was almost certain to introduce infection, so often fatal.[3]

Dobbie's characterization of Mother Nature "failing in her task" in the context of bumbling early modern midwives is, in itself, fodder for a rich discussion of gender and contemporary gynecological rhetoric about the past. While that metacritical study is not the focus here, it does serve to contextualize the work of McTavish and others who seek to put into question the assumptions that such characterizations validate. To be sure, however, Dobbie's suppositions participate fully in the highly gendered discourse of this era that François Rouget and Colette Winn describe as clearly polemic:

> C'est dans le dernier tiers du XVIe siècle que s'amorce le fameux conflit entre les practiciennes et les "hommes d'art" opposant les femmes, fortes de leur experience mais ignorantes des principes élémentaires de l'anatomie et de l'hygiène, qui refusaient de céder le monopole dont elles avaient joui jusque-là dans le domaine obstetrical, aux hommes, qui souvent n'avaient qu'une connaissance théorique des mécanismes de la parturition.[4]
>
> [It is in the final third part of the sixteenth century that begins the famous conflict between female practitioners and the "men of medical arts" opposing these women who were fortified by their experience but ignorant of basic principles of anatomy and hygiene and refused to give up the monopoly they had theretofore enjoyed in the realm of obstetrics over men who often had only theoretical knowledge of the mechanics of birthing.]

Of concern to me here are the ways in which anxiety over the woman's body in birth inflects this polarized debate. Rouget and Winn continue: "Le respect des traditions mais aussi les préjugés et les tabous, notamment la pudeur et la peur qu'avaient les femmes d'être souillée, ne cessaient d'alimenter le fameux débat sur 'l'indécence aux hommes d'accoucher les femmes'" [Respect for tradition but also prejudices and taboos, notably modesty and women's fear of being sullied, did not cease from fueling the infamous debate on the "indecency of

---

[3] B.M. Willmott Dobbie, "An Attempt to Estimate the True Rate of Maternal Mortality, Sixteenth to Eighteenth Centuries," *Medical History*, 26 (1982): p. 79.

[4] François Rouget and Colette Winn, "Introduction" to Louise Boursier, *Récit veritable de la naissance de messeigneurs et dames les enfans de France; Instruction à ma fille et autres textes* (Geneva, 2000), p. 16. All translations are my own unless otherwise noted.

men assisting women in childbirth"] (17). If Dobbie raises the specter of well-intentioned birth attendants "fumbling in the dark," so do I here take up the veiled and anxious discourse around who is privileged to fumble about; how early modern birth attendants approached their mission; and how their writing defended their decisions and livelihood. Not surprisingly, Louise Boursier, whom Wendy Perkins hails as "the foremost female health worker in France," plays a crucial role here.[5] Having compared Boursier's account of the birth of the future Louis XIII with Gargantua in the previous chapter, I now propose to put her *Récits d'accouchement* into dialogue with other, more medically inspired sources, to tell a different story about women, men, and control over the birthing body. Midwife to the Parisian elite of her day, including, on six occasions, Marie de Médicis, Boursier sets the scene in her *Observations diverses* of 1609:

> … je me trouvais un jour à l'accouchement d'une honnête demoiselle de mes bonnes amies, de laquelle le mari était absent; elle était assistée de trois ou quatre de ses amies, lesquelles me demandèrent l'état de son accouchement, je leur dis que l'enfant venait mal, mais que je l'aurais, aidant Dieu, sans danger de la mère ni de l'enfant; elles me prièrent d'avoir agréable de la faire voir au chirurgien; pour leur décharge, je leur accordai, pourvu qu'elle ne le vît point, d'autant que je savais que cela était capable de la faire mourir d'appréhension, et de honte. Je la persuadai de se glisser aux pieds de son lit. Je mis le chevet au milieu du lit et abattis le tour du lit du côté qu'il devait passer, et aux pieds: il la toucha comme je parlais, elle ne le vit point, et accoucha sans artifice ni aide, que de Dieu et de la nature.[6]
>
> [… I found myself one day at the birthing of a proper lady known to my good friends whose husband was absent; she was attended to by three or four of her friends who asked me about the progress of the birth. I told them that the child was coming with difficulty but that I would receive it, God willing, without danger to the mother or to the child; they asked me kindly if I would consent to having her seen by a surgeon; to assuage their fears, I consented, provided that she not be allowed to see him, for I knew that this could cause her to die of apprehension or shame. I persuaded her to slide to the foot of the bed. I put the pillow in the middle and built up the bed on the side where he would approach, as well as down by her feet. He touched her while I spoke; she never

[5] "Between 1601 and 1609 she was midwife to Marie de Médicis, queen of France, delivering all six of her children. Her rise to prominence was in fact meteoric: having passed the official examination only in 1598, she had by 1601 delivered the future Louis XIII and was assured of a successful, influential career." Wendy Perkins, *Midwifery and Medicine in Early Modern France: Louise Bourgeois* (Exeter, 1996), p. 1.

[6] Louise Boursier, *Observations diverses sur la stérilité, perte de fruict, accouchements, et maladies des femmes, et enfants nouveaux naiz*, ed. Françoise Olive (Paris, 1992), p. 187.

> laid eyes on him and gave birth without any special intervention or help, either from God or nature.]

Such anecdotes are one of the most compelling features of the midwife's or physician's manual. Nestled in among Petrarchan sonnetry in the dedications, classical and folkloric allusions, herbal remedies and tips on everything from dry skin and vomiting to paternity and multiple births, the eyewitness account is what turns the pages. *I saw, I attended, I saved.* These are the terms that lend respect and veracity. Boursier's story here is a particularly poignant one for what it says about the state of the increasingly medicalized view of childbirth for women of elevated social standing. It betrays the moment where attending to women's reproduction and birthing was literally slipping from the midwife's hands.[7]

Boursier's narrative is couched clearly in an atmosphere of mistrust regarding women's capacities to oversee births, particularly in the case of difficult ones. In consenting to her client's wishes to have a doctor present, she must stage an elaborate deception so that the birthing woman hears her, but is touched by the man behind the screen: "il la toucha comme je parlais, elle ne le vit point, et accoucha sans artifice ni aide, que de Dieu et de la nature" [He touched her while I spoke; she never laid eyes on him and gave birth without any special intervention or help, either from God or nature]. She talks reassuringly and he touches. Boursier, related as she was through marriage to some of the most renowned surgeons of her day, is not overly begrudging; but we do sense in the "sans artifice ni aide"—meaning that no extraordinary measures were needed that would have required a doctor—that this was something that could have been handled (pun intended) between women. Louise Boursier reminds her daughter and the reader in her *Instruction à ma fille* that her confidence as a medical professional is linked both to a pantheon of ancient midwives and to the combined knowledge of her entire family, whose members are engaged in medical practice (see Chapter 2).[8] Louise

[7] Of insight in this realm of investigation, particularly with regard to the example of Louise Boursier, is Wendy Perkins's study, *Midwifery and Medicine in Early Modern France*; Rouget and Winn's edition of Boursier's *Récit véritable* is highly useful with regard to primary work by Boursier and biography. Of interest as well is the more universal study of women and medicine by Evelyne Berriot-Salvadore, *Un Corps, un Destin: La femme dans la médecine de la Renaissance* (Paris, 1993).

[8] Boursier writes, "Advisez ma fille, ce que vous pouvez estre plus que moy: estant petite fille de Phanerote, disciple de Lucine, maistresse de Mercure, à cause que Lucine l'a assujetty à vostre mere. Vous estes née dans l'exercice que ceste sage m'a monstré … Vous n'en manquerez nullement, d'autant que vous estes enfant de famille, un Docteur en medecine est mary de vostre soeur, vostre mary fait son cours pour l'estre, l'un de vos freres est Pharmacien, vostre pere est Chirurgien, et moy sage-femme; le corps de la medecine est entier dans nostre maison." [Consider, my daughter, that you can become even greater than I: being granddaughter of Phanerote, disciple of Lucina, mistress of Mercury because Lucina put her in your mother's service. You are born into the work that this wise woman showed me … You can't hardly fail, being a child in such a family, your sister's husband

Boursier's husband, Martin Boursier, studied under Ambroise Paré and became one of the king's surgeons. Boursier indulges both her actual lineage so redolent of medical acumen and, more importantly, her female mythological forbearers, whom she uses to establish her credibility as a midwife. And for good reason, it would appear.

Professional medical men were increasingly implicating themselves into the process of childbirth; the written record of their advice regarding their profession reflects not only the fact of their involvement, but a certain anxiety regarding the tensions between men and women, surgeons and midwives, that clearly marked this period of transition.[9] One can explore more closely this phenomenon through a shared narrative, a story taken up by the surgeon Jacques Guillemeau in his *De l'Heureux accouchement des femmes* of 1609 and interpreted differently by another writer with more literary pretentions, Catherine des Roches, in her first published works, *Les Oeuvres*, of 1579. The story that both retell is that of Agnodice, the mythic first woman physician who attended to the women of Athens, fearful for their reputations lest they be seen and touched by men. The story came to both authors through Hyginus, a second-century Latinist as published in his *Fabulae*. Their respective approaches to this tale are the stuff of gendered authorship: What do they include? Why? Who constitutes their putative readership? What is at stake?

Hyginus and (Women's) Hygiene

Hyginus embeds his story in a chapter entitled "Inventors and their Inventions" wherein a variety of discoveries and inventions are discussed: wine, pruning, the

---

is a doctor of medicine, your own husband is studying to be one, one of your brothers is a pharmacist, your father is a surgeon, and I, a midwife; the entire medical establishment is represented in our household.] *Instruction à ma fille*, in Rouget and Winn, *Récit veritable*, p. 124.

[9] Of primary importance to this discussion—and of some help in my conception of a title for this chapter—is the work of Caroline Bicks on Shakespearean midwives: "What distinguishes the early modern midwife from the other women of the birthroom, however, is the fact that she was recognized as a sanctioned shaper of men's, women's, and children's bodies. Although any birth attendant was theoretically privy to a new mother's secrets, the midwife had an acknowledged duty to handle bodies and interpret their secrets. Given that European men had participated in making the midwife an integral part of their countries' institutional structures and less tangible cultural operations, her tales and touch posed a particular challenge to male claims about women's bodies and children's origins—and to the masculine identities that those claims helped underwrite." Caroline Bicks, *Midwiving Subjects in Shakespeare's England* (Aldershot, 2003), p. 12). See also Lianne McTavish's cautionary interpretation of this issue as discussed in my introduction, where she warns against an overly polemicized debate according to gender.

needle, bronze, lead, arms, and then somewhat incongruously, herbs, which lead to a reference to Chiron, son of Saturn (first to use herbs in the medical art of surgery), Apollo (first to practice in the art of treating eyes), and his son Asclepius, who purportedly began the art of clinical medicine. The story of Agnodice follows:

> The ancients didn't have obstetricians, and as a result, women because of modesty perished. For the Athenians forbade slaves and women to learn the art of medicine. A certain girl, Hagnodice, virgin, desired to learn medicine, and since she desired it, she cut her hair, and in male attire came to a certain Herophilus for training. When she had learned the art, and had heard that a woman was in labor, she came to her. And when the woman refused to trust herself to her, thinking that she was a man, she removed her garment to show that she was a woman, and in this way she treated women. When the doctors saw that they were not admitted to women, they began to accuse Hagnodice, saying that "he" was a seducer and corruptor of women, and that the women were pretending to be ill. The Areopagites, in session, started to condemn Hagnodice, but Hagnodice removed her garment for them and showed that she was a woman. Then the doctors began to accuse her more vigorously, and as a result the leading women came to the Court and said: "You are not husbands, but enemies, because you condemn her who discovered safety for us." Then the Athenians amended the law, so that free-born women could learn the art of medicine.[10]

Hyginus then quite characteristically shifts gears and plunges straight away into a list of other inventions: compasses, statuary, astrology, dye, musical pipes, and so forth. This "invention," as it were, is far more elaborated than any other items in Hyginus's chapter; it seems to carry a lot more weight. His attention betrays a conscious and concerted attention to the issue of women's health and the anxieties attached to it. Hyginus introduces this "invention" or origin story as being about female obstetricians. Yet it is curious to note how he has the Athenian women characterize it within his narrative: "You are not

[10] Hyginus, *The Myths of Hyginus*, ed. and trans. Mary Grant (Lawrence, 1960). The identity of the author Hyginus remains subject to ardent debate. Mary Grant seems clear that he was not the commonly accepted C. Julius Hyginus, freedman of Augustus and librarian of the Palatine Library, but paints an ample portrait of the author, based upon evidence from the text itself and contemporary sources. The recent French edition, edited by Jean-Yves Boriaud (Paris, 2003), still accepts this attribution of Hyginus as a learned freedman, friend of Ovid, erudite and close to the seats of power in contrast to Grant (relying heavily on H.J. Rose's critical edition), who sees evidence in this early work of little more than "a mere schoolboy, and not a very alert one at that" (Grant, p. 3). In any case, it appears clear that the text of the *Fabulae* (known in the original, presumably, as *Genealogiae*) was a type of reference for writers wishing to utilize Greek and Roman myths in some way (Grant, p. 4).

husbands, but enemies, because you condemn her who discovered safety for us" [Vos coniuges non estis sed hostes, quia quae *salutem* nobis inuenit eam damnatis].[11] In a gesture reminiscent of Aristophanes's *Lysistrata*, where sex is withheld for peace, the Greek women rise up and command the patriarchy into submission; the drama of their proclamation mirrors the drama of the central acts of disrobing and discovery. It is not hard to see the connections to the anxieties of covering, uncovering ("illa tunica sublata ostendebat se feminam esse" and "tunicam alleuauit et se ostendit feminam esse"), hiding and revealing, suffering and healing so crucial to the story I began with by Louise Boursier.

Of particular relevance to this investigation is the thoroughgoing work of Helen King, whose study of the historical Agnodice (Agnodike to this Hellenist) focuses heavily on the act of "anasyrmos," the gesture of lifting of the garments to reveal the lower part of the body.[12] King shows this gesture to be highly charged and enumerates its many meanings: whether to drive away evil forces, to invite fertility, to provoke laughter, to make oneself sexually available, to shame men in retreat in battle, to prove one's sexual identity, or, as in the case among women, to show solidarity. For the purposes of this study, it is these latter two impulses that take precedence, though the wartime scenario—literally, "Is this where you cowards are running back to, back to your mother's womb?"—has some poignancy if we remind ourselves again of Aristophanes's *Lysistrata*, in which women's sexual power is wielded with remarkable, transformative effect, though presumably to opposite ends. King aptly remarks the context in which the story of Agnodice is told: Hyginus's "quis quid inuenerit"—more literally, who discovered what—with an emphasis on *covering* and *un-covering*. To find out how this was played out in early modern France, we turn first to physician Jacques Guillemeau.

A Surgeon's Handling of Hyginus

Guillemeau's retelling of Hyginus is included at the beginning of Book II of his medical treatise, wherein he devotes 13 pages to the duties of midwives (the entire book is 200 pages long). If the percentage of time spent on women's role as practitioners at childbirth is relatively small, it might be explained in the rhetoric of danger and precariousness with which he approaches his subject:

> Or comme ainsi soit que la plus grande maladie que les femmes puissent avoir, est celle des neuf mois, dont la crise & guarison se faict par leur accouchement:

[11] English translation, Grant, Hyginus, p. 176; Latin original, Hyginus, *Fabulae*, ed. Peter K. Marshall (Munich, 2002), pp. 196–7.

[12] Helen King, "Agnodike and the Profession of Medicine," *Proceedings of the Cambridge Philological Society*, 32 (1986): pp. 53–77.

> Il ne faut point douter que telles femmes ne se soient addonnees & exercees aux accouchemens des femmes, & qu'il y en a eu de tout temps.[13]
>
> [Now since the greatest disease that women can have is that of the nine Moneths, the Crisis and cure whereof consists in their safe deliverie: we must not doubt, but that there have been some women addicted thereto, and practized therein, in all ages.][14]

The audience is clearly marked as the fraternity of surgeons who must come to terms with the sorority of midwives, as it were, "addonnee & exercees" to the work that men were gradually taking over.

Guillemeau retells the story with clear emphasis on the crisis in women's health:

> ...la necessité, maistresse des arts, a contrainct les femmes, les unes avec les autres d'apprendre & practiquer la Medecine: car se trouvans affligees & atteintes de plusieurs maladies en leurs parties honteuses, estans destituees de tous remedes: à faute de quoy plusieurs languissoient, & mouroient miserablement, n'ont osé se descouvrir, & deceler leur mal, qu'à elles-mesmes estimans cela deshonneste. (Guillemeau, *De l'Heureux accouchement* 143–4)
>
> [necessitie, (the mistresse of Arts) hath constrained women, to learne and practise Physicke, one with an other. For finding themselves afflicted, and troubled with divers diseases in their naturall parts, and being destitute of all remedies, (for want whereof many perished, and died miserably) they durst not discover, and lay open their infirmities, to any but themselves, accounting it to be dishonest.] (*Child-birth* 80)

It is not surprising that Hyginus's characterization of women "perishing for modesty" came to mind. The "discovering" and "laying open" here of infirmities is clearly related to women's genitalia, the site of childbirth, to be sure; but also of intercourse, desire, shame, pollution, and the ever-threatening licentiousness of women's exposed bodies—the "parties honteuses"—to which we will shall return. Guillemeau's version sticks closely to the myth as told by Hyginus; his is a fairly faithful rendering of the tightly constructed drama of Agnodice's desire for learning: the physical transformation of her hair and clothes; her uncovering of herself to the doubting Athenian women; her subsequent development of an enthusiastic following; the Athenian men's accusation of transvestism and debauchery—ironically that she

[13] Jacques Guillemeau, *De l'Heureux accouchement des femmes, où il est traicté du gouvernement de leur grossesse, de leur travail naturel et contre nature; du traictement es tant accouchées et de leurs maladies* (Paris, 1609), p. 146.

[14] Jacques Guillemeau, *Child-birth or, The Happy Deliverie of Women*, anonymous translation (London, 1612), p. 81.

might be a man posing as a woman; the second "discovery" as her raised tunic proves them wrong; the charge of greater concern, that of studying and practicing as a woman; the Athenian women's uprising and condemnation of the men's objections; and finally, the revising of Athenian law to allow women to study medicine.

Two discrepancies are noticeable and significant. First, it is telling that in Guillemeau's version, Agnodice is said to return from medical school (as it were) to practice first upon a woman characterized as "afflicted in her shameful parts": "ayant esté advertie qu'il y avoit quelque femme *malade en ses parties honteuses*, alla vers elle, pour luy offrir son service: Ce que la malade recusa [sic], estimant que ce fust un homme" (Guillemeau 144, my emphasis) [having notice of a certaine woman that *was troubled in her naturall parts*; she went unto her, and made proffer of her service; which the sicke party refused, thinking she had been a man] (*Child-birth* 80). This is indeed how he introduced the idea of midwifery: a profession born out of women's shame. Hyginus's description of Agnodice's first client was, we may remember, unattached to shame ("et feminam *laborantem audisset ab inferiore parte*"); the "laborantem" does not necessarily suggest the labor of childbirth, as would "parturire." Yet it is somewhat ironic that it would suggest, indeed, "suffering under bodily affliction," but also "a state of being troubled or anxious"; in this case, Guillemeau is seen layering the narrative with the specter of shame and embarrassment more with respect to *himself* than to the woman. Guillemeau appears too troubled or anxious to call it like it is—this "inferiore parte"—without invoking the shamefulness of the woman's vagina and uterus.

Interesting as well is the way in which the two authors describe the climax of the story wherein the Athenian women speak out against the unreasonable injunctions against women's participation in medicine. From Hyginus, who gives them direct speech: "'You are not husbands, but enemies, because you condemn her who discovered safety for us'" (Grant 176) ["Vos coniuges non estis sed hostes, quia quae salutem nobis inuenit eam damnatis"] (Marshall 197); and from Guillemeau: "qu'elles ne les tenoient aucunement pour leurs maris & amis, mais pour ennemis, de vouloir condamner celle qui leur donnoit la santé" (Guillemeau 145) ["that they did not account them, for their husbands, and friends, but for enemies; that they would condemne her, which restor'd them to their health"] (*Child-birth* 80). Hyginus tells his story in the context of inventors and inventions, people who discover. Agnodice is therefore the actor, the discoverer, the first woman gynecologist, who invents women's safety. Hyginus's women's speech is direct; Guillemeau's is reported. Guillemeau's text remains one about healing and restoring health, a medical view of everything pertaining to women's well-being; the intensity of the Athenian women's dramatic declaration is diminished by the indirect discourse, their voices silenced. Agnodice remains in some ways transvested for Guillemeau. He makes no plea for changes in the laws of early modern France to allow women to practice medicine; for all of the drama that the transvesting narrative affords, Guillemeau's tale is not meant to empower women to become doctors, but to remind men, the "we" in his text (the ubiquitous and unquestionably masculine "on"), that women may well continue to lay claim to this burgeoning profession.[15]

All the better, the reader might well surmise, from the description of bedside fumbling about in the dark that he describes in his "Au Lecteur":

> Or pour la dexterité, il n'y a rien de comparaison avec les autres o[pe]rations: car il ne se faict aucunes oeuvres en Chirurgie, où il ne soit necessaire de voir clair, soit par la lumiere, qui nous est donnee du jour, ou de la chandelle, & que la partie que l'on traicte & manie, ne soit apparente & manifeste à l'oeil. Au contraire, en ceste operation, tant pour la presence de ceux qui assistent, que pour la crainte que pourroit avoir la femme, l'on est contrainct de cacher seulement l'entrée par laquelle il faut mettre la main, puis icelle y estant mise, il faut chercher l'enfant en quelque situation qu'il soit, sans le pouvoir voir … (Guillemeau, e i)
>
> [Now for the dexteritie: there is no comparision betweene this and other practises; for there be no workes to be done in Chirurgery; where it is not necessary, to have the benefit either of daylight or candle light, and the part which is to be handled, and dressed must be apparent and laid open to the eye. Whereas contrariwise in this worke as well by reason of the company present, as also, least the woman should be afraid, the very entrance, whereby hee should put in his hand, they are constrained to hide: and then his hand being there, he must search for the child (howsoever it be placed) not being able to see it.] (*Child-birth* 7b)

Guillemeau's text suggests the challenge of men practicing on women in a society fearful of women's exposure or discovery in public: here we have the physician's version of what it was like to attend to a birth such as the one described by Louise Boursier from the beginning of this chapter; Guillemeau betrays the compromised nature of this fumbling delivery himself. There is nowhere to look without fear or shame, and yet Guillemeau bravely flounts the social proscriptions, reaches in and touches, delivers. Tellingly, while Guillemeau is often suspicious of midwives' competency in their vocation because of their gender, he does bring them on the scene in his manual when it comes to the "internal exam" to verify pregnancy:

> … un signe aussi bien certain est recogneu par la Sage-femme, en mettant son doigt dedans le col de la matrice, duquel elle touchera le col interieur d'icelle:

[15] For a contemporaneous example of the battle of the sexes and professions that was played out in print, one need only consult the reports of surgeons regarding the death of Marie de Bourbon Montpensier, five days after giving birth while attended by Louise Boursier (see Chapter 1). The report implicates Louise Boursier as negligent, a charge to which she replies in her *Fidelle relation de l'accouchement, maladie et ouverture du corps de feu MADAME*. For both see Rouget and Winn's modern edition of Boursier's *Récit véritable*, Appendices I and II, pp. 97–120.

> si la femme est grosse, elle la trouvera si exactement fermee, que la pointe d'une esguille n'y pourroit pas entrer, il sera mollet neantmoins, & sans estre accompagné d'aucune dureté, lequel pareillement sera retiré en haut, s'estant raccourcy retroussé à raison du corps de la matrice qui s'est resserree en soy, pour embrasser la semence, ce qui est cause que ladite Sage-femme n'y peut toucher que difficilement. (Guillemeau 10)

> [... another certaine signe may be perceived by the Midwife, who putting up her finger into the wombe to touch the inner orifice thereof, if the woman be with child she shall finde it so close shut, that the point of a needle will scarse enter therein, yet soft, and without any hardnesse, which also will bee drawn upward being shrunke and as it were trussed up, because the body of the Matrice doth gather it selfe together to embrace the seed, which is the reason that the Midwife can very hardly come to reach it with her finger.] (*Child-birth* 7)

Such intimate knowledge of the woman's cervix is best recounted, it would appear, with a woman's probing finger in mind. What Guillemeau argues for, ever so circuitously here, is safer delivery. His rhetoric of "shameful parts," however, suggests that while the birth of the child may be inevitable, the birth of truly enlightened knowledge and safety regarding women's reproduction may be a ways off.

Agnodice as Medical and Literary Gyn-Ecologist

Turning to Catherine des Roches's retelling of the myth of Agnodice, one finds illuminating counterpoint. Inserted in a poetic collection whose themes betray an enthusiastic appraisal of women's community and their literary and domestic lives, this Agnodice becomes a touchstone for women's health and knowability in a way far beyond the scope of Guillemeau.

Catherine des Roches is no physician; she is, however, in the more generous and radical sense of the term, an avid gyn-ecologist (with thanks to Mary Daly).[16] Her version of the Agnodice myth appears in the context of a woman writer coming to terms with bodies of writing, writing bodies, and all of the rich attendant allusions to safety, patriarchal control, and sisterhood that we have observed so far in Louise Boursier and Jacques Guillemeau. Her Agnodice is told by an author who has eschewed births of living children in favor of children of the spirit. As she says to her mother in the preface to the volume that includes the Agnodice (and which I develop in my introduction):

---

[16] The radical connection that Mary Daly makes in her groundbreaking work between women's physical and intellectual and spiritual health is most pertinent to this discussion (see Introduction). See Mary Daly, *Gyn/Ecology: The Metaethics of Radical Feminism* (Boston, MA, 1978).

> J'ay seulement pensé de vous monstrer comme j'employe le temps de ma plus grande oisiveté, et vous supplie humblement (ma mere) de recevoir ces petits escrits qui vous en rendront tesmoignage; si vous en trouvez quelques-uns qui soient assez bien nez, avoüez-les s'il vous plaist pour voz nepveux, et ceux qui ne vous seront agreables, punissez-les à l'exemple de Jacob qui condemna la famille d'Isachar pour obeir à ses autres enfans.
>
> [I have only thought of showing you how I employ my idle time, and humbly beseech you (my Mother) to receive this little collection of writing that bears witness to you; if you find some of them well enough conceived, please acknowledge them as your very own progeny, and those that you do not find agreeable, punish them in the same way Jacob condemned the family of Issachar to serve his other children.][17]

Catherine des Roches presents her writings to her own mother as the fruits of her scholarly labor. The "nepveux" of whom she speaks is a play on her mother's birth name, Neveu, felicitously combined with the latinate *neveux* (from *nepotes*) or descendants.[18] What Catherine des Roches gives birth to is a broad-ranging collection of dialogues, sonnets, occasional poems, dedications, epitaphs, a theatrical piece, and the retelling of several biblical and mythological tales. It is a large family she has spawned. The favorite daughter, for my purposes here, is her 177-line verse rendition of the tale of Agnodice.

Her mother, Madeleine des Roches, has previously shown herself predisposed to literary rather than flesh-and-blood grandchildren; indeed her Ode 1, included in this joint publication, presents one of the most unglamorous and cranky diatribes against wedlock and motherhood one could imagine:

> Noz parens ont de loüables coustumes,
> Pour nous tollir l'usage de raison,
> De nous tenir closes dans la maison
> Et nous donner le fuzeau pour la plume.
>
> Trassant noz pas selon la destinée,
> On nous promet liberté et plaisir:
> Et nous payons l'obstiné desplaisir,
> Portant le dot sous les loix d'Hymenée.

---

[17] Catherine des Roches, *Les Oeuvres* (1579), ed. Anne R. Larsen (Geneva, 1993), p. 185. Translation: Anne R. Larsen: *From Mother and Daughter: poems, dialogues, and letters of les dames des Roches/Madeleine and Catherine des Roches* (Chicago, 2006), p. 87. All references to and translations of this work are taken from Larsen's *From Mother and Daughter*.

[18] See Larsen's edition of *Les Oeuvres*, p. 185, n. 11.

Bientost apres survient une misere
Qui naist en nous d'un desir mutuel,
Accompagné d'un soing continuel,
Qui suit tousjours l'entraille de la mere.

[Our parents have laudable customs
To deprive us of the use of our reason:
They lock us up at home
And hand us the spindle instead of the pen

Conforming our steps to our (female) destiny,
They promise us liberty and pleasure:
But we reap continuous displeasure,
When we lose our dowry to the laws of Marriage.

Then soon after comes a new misery,
Born within us of mutual desire,
Accompanied by those continuous cares
That always burden the mother's womb.] (53)

Real progeny seem like the end of a raw deal, wherein bright women are robbed of their study time (giving up the pen for the distaff, an image that her daughter will take up directly in her poem "A ma quenoille") and burdened with the inequitable rules and duties of marriage. One might imagine a far warmer depiction of the arrival of a child than her "misere/qui naist en nous d'un desir mutuel" followed by constant worry by a mother reduced to a burdened gut. One might also imagine a more tempered depiction, given the embeddedness of her poem within the works of her very own, cherished daughter; history suggests however, that Catherine was fully aware of the hardships of the married, childbearing life, a path she chose to avoid—to the bafflement and consternation of a multitude of suitors, but not, presumably, of her mother.[19]

---

[19] See the judgments of the family friend Estienne Pasquier as he ruminates over Catherine des Roches's reticence in matters of marriage: "Il n'y a qu'une chose qui me déplaise en ceste maison, qu'estant la fille belle en perfection tant de corps que d'esprit, riche de biens, comme celle qui doit estre l'unique heritiere de sa mere, requise en mariage par une infinité de personnages d'honneur, toutes-fois elle met toutes ces requestes sous pied; resolue de vivre & mourir avec sa mère" [There is but one thing that displeases me in this household, that the daughter, possessed of a perfect beauty of both body and soul, wealthy (as she is her mother's sole inheritor), all the same, she refuses all suitors, resolved to live and die with her mother]. Estienne Pasquier, *Letter to Monsieur Pithou, Seigneur de Savoye* (Book VI, Letter 11 of his *Lettres familières*), in Anne R. Larsen's edition of Madeleine and Catherine des Roches, *Les Missives* (1586) (Geneva, 1999), pp. 348–9.

Who then, does Agnodice become for Catherine des Roches? Agnodice arrives as a stranger to rescue the Athenian women who are condemned to a life robbed of learning as a consequence of the death of Phocion and the anger of Envy. Envy induces all husbands to become tyrants, forbidding their wives to read books, thereby sapping them of the desire or force of will to live. To one such victim she growls:

> "Car en despit de toy j'animeray les ames 61
> Des maris, qui seront les tyrans de leurs femmes,
> Et qui leur deffendant le livre et le sçavoir,
> Leur osteront aussi de vivre le pouvoir."
>
> ["For to spite you, I'll incite
> Husbands to become the tyrants of their wives;
> By keeping learning and books from them,
> They'll take away their very desire to live."] (124–5)

Des Roches thus embellishes the Hyginus tale at the onset by positing the source of women's torment, not as the pangs of labor, or the onset of some gynecological disorder, but as a physical reaction to the privation of their vocational, or better, literary aspirations. The decree causes a physical malaise that soon afflicts the spiritually bereft women:

> Les dames aussitost se trouverent suivies 73
> De fiebvres, de langueurs, et d'autres maladies;
> Leur faisoit supporter incroyables tourmens.
> Aymant trop mieux mourir que d'estre peu honteuses 76
> Contant aux Medecins leurs peines langoureuses,
> Les femmes (o pitié!) n'osoient plus se mesler
> De s'aider l'une l'autre; on les faisoit filler.
>
> [The women soon found themselves beset
> By fevers, faintness, and other illnesses,
> Envy forced them to bear incredible torments.
> They preferred death to the shame of
> Telling the [male] Doctors about their debilitating troubles.
> The women (what a pity!) did not dare
> To help one another, they were made to spin.] (126–7)

The "tourmens" and "peines langoureuses" are quite clearly references to the women-and-knowledge boilerplate text from Genesis, that the torments of labor are a reminder of woman's original sin, the sin of desire for knowledge whose consequences are likewise linked to her reproductive capacities.

Enter Agnodice.

Ceste Dame, cachant l'or de sa blonde tresse
Aprist la medecine, et s'en feit grand maistresse.
Puis se resouvenant de son affection,
Voulut effectuer sa bonne intention,
Et guerir les douleurs de ses pauvres voisines

[This young woman, hiding the gold of her blond locks,
Learned medicine, and became quite expert at it.
Then, remembering her original intent,
She wanted to carry out her plan
To heal the sufferings of her poor sisters] (126–7)

Agnodice returns and the crucial scene "self-disclosure" or "self-discovery" is enacted:

Agnodice, voyant leur grande chasteté,
Les estima beaucoup pour ceste honnesteté;
Lors descouvrant du sein les blanches pommes rondes,
Et de son chef doré les belles tresses blondes,
Monstre qu'elle estoit fille, et que son gentil cueur
Les vouloit delivrer de leur triste langueur.
Les Dames admirant ceste honte naïsve,
Et de son teint douillet la blanche couleur vive,
Et de son sein poupin le petit mont jumeau,
Et de son chef sacré l'or crepelu tant beau,
Et de ses yeux divins les flammes ravissantes,
Et de ses doux propos les graces attirantes,
Baiserent mille fois et sa bouche et son sein,
Recevant le secours de son heureuse main.

[Agnodice, seeing their great chastity,
Esteemed them all the more for their virtue,
And uncovering then the white round apples (of her bosom),
And the beautiful blond tresses of her golden head,
Showed that she was a maiden, and that her kind heart
Wished to deliver them from their sad predicament.
The Ladies admiring her innocent modesty,
And the lively whiteness of her soft complexion,
And the little twin mounts of her adorable breasts,
And the beautiful golden shine of her blessed head,
And the ravishing flames of her divine eyes,
And the engaging gracefulness of her sweet words,
Kissed a thousand times both her mouth and her breast,
As they received help from her blessed hands.] (127, 129)

The story here becomes ever more lyrical, ecstatic, and erotic; the women of Athens are delivered from their "langueur"—the illness induced by the privation of learning—into a state of delirious contentment. In contrast to Hyginus and Guillemeau (and most poignantly, perhaps, to Boursier), the woman's body is touchable, and knowable in a way that flies in the face of accusations of licentiousness: des Roches participates fully in the rhetoric of love poetry, and of the blazon in particular as she delineates the woman's body in all its glorious detail. She lingers specifically on the breast, "les blanches pommes rondes" [the white round apples] reiterated in "son sein poupin le petit mont jumeau" [the little twin mounts of her adorable breasts] illuminated by the "flammes ravissantes" [ravishing flames] of her heavenly countenance. The scene culminates in rapture as the Athenian women kiss her mouth and breast while receiving the help of her blessed hand.

Other possible illusions from the ancient world attest ever more suggestively to a view to women's empowerment and community. In Greek myth, Baubo, in an attempt to relieve the torment of grief, was said to have joked with the bereaved goddess Demeter by painting a face on her stomach and then pulling her dress over her head and dancing. The anger and anguish that the Athenian women express is clearly fueled by grief over their neglected sisters. The sisterhood of the goddess Diana surrounded by her nymphs is clearly another reference, especially given the physical descriptions: Diana is the chaste female figure *par excellence*, whose very existence relied on the exclusion of men for their survival (and when you got too close, you got eaten by your own dogs …). Helen King remarks this possible allusion to the original Agnodice, placing it squarely in the context of Hyginus's work. In Fabula 189, he retells the story of Procris, a woman, who cuts her hair and dons a tunic and challenges and beats her husband in a hunt. He asks for the javelin and the dog that Diana had given her in exchange for money; she asks instead for sex and reveals herself posthaste as a woman: "tunicam leuauit et ostendit se feminam esse et coniugem eius" (King 61). The utopian gynaceum that des Roches depicts is rich with the erotic potential of her ancient predecessors, here to the exclusion of men.

Such a contrast we have here to the plight of Guillemeau, whose *unhappy* hand gropes about blindly in the dark, ashamed both for himself and for his patient. Des Roches's women, on the other hand, have found not only health and safety, but a renaissance in letters rendered through this particular climactic moment, an act that would be impossible, inappropriate, indeed unspeakable, by Agnodice's male counterpart. Agnodice arrives and is given this excited welcome by women thanks to the fact that they have at last a healer who, with no sense of impropriety or shame, can touch them. When word gets around that Agnodice is attending to these women to their obvious well-being and delight, the same scene of revelation is enacted for the male authorities who, in a fantasy of stunning conversion, stand in mute, awed acceptance:

> Depuis qu'elle eut parlé, oncq une seulle voix
> Ne s'esleva contre elle; ains toute l'assistance

> Monstroit d'esmerveiller ceste rare excellence;
> Ils estoient tous ravis, sans parler ny mouvoir,
> Ententifs seulement à l'ouyr et la voir.
> Comme l'on voit parfois apres un long orage,
> R'asserener les vents, et calmer le ravage …
>
> [After she had spoken, not a single voice
> Was raised against her; on the contrary, the entire audience
> Marveled at her rare excellence;
> Everyone was filled with wonder, and no one moved or made a sound,
> Attentive only to hearing and seeing her.
> In like manner one sometimes sees, after a long storm,
> The winds die down, and the waves become calm.] (131)

And so Catherine des Roches dispenses with the scene wherein Agnodice is condemned and then subsequently defended by her Athenian sisters; in her version, Agnodice's compelling oratory on her own behalf stuns the men into submission. The storm of controversy surrounding women attending to women is calmed entirely by one learned and persuasive woman. Agnodice singlehandedly transforms the Envy-tainted society that has banished women from books and learning and begins the work of repairing wounded minds and bodies. Agnodice is the midwife of children of both the body and the spirit. The labor is difficult and noble and cherished for women in a society suspicious and highly proscriptive, a society that links women's unworthiness constantly to the messiness, the shame, and the mutable nature of their bodies. And so Agnodice arrives to dispel such mythologizing and indeed to turn such opinion on its head: perhaps women are worthy and capable *because* of this ability to reproduce.

Facing the Blank Page and Women's Reproductivity

I hope to have demonstrated that the retelling of the myth of Agnodice by a physician, Jacques Guillemeau, and an early modern female poet, Catherine des Roches, means different things for the authors and constituencies concerned. Guillemeau's version is retold in the context of a sincere coming-to-terms with the anxieties and exigencies surrounding women's health at the time; he is not immune to the illogical, silly, and ultimately dangerous proscriptions against men's "illumination" with regard to women's health—he does not use the tale of Agnodice, however, to propose education for women that would allow them to take over his role. He is interested in producing responsible midwives who know when to call the doctor. Catherine des Roches, on the other hand, extols the glories of women as at once (re)producers, midwives, and physicians as a metaphor for protecting women's livelihood in the realm of letters. Their ecstatic enthusiasm comes in equal measure to the immense oppression we saw quite clearly and sadly drawn in her mother's first ode.

To conclude, I would direct us to a document of keen interest to this discussion from a contemporaneous translation of Guillemeau's text. It is the anonymous translator's epistle wherein he feels compelled to defend himself for having brought such delicate material to light. It is he who makes the most eloquent bridge between literary and anatomical production one could imagine. His anxiety is everywhere apparent:

> Thus far hath the Authour pleaded for him selfe, whom while I Translate, least the fault be translated upon me, I will speake somewhat for my selfe, before I be accused: least when I am accused, there be no bodie to speake for me: If therefore it be thought prejudiciall, either to the literarie common-wealth of *Physicke*, that I have exported and made common a commoditie, which the learned would have had private to themselves: or if I have been offensive to Women, in prostituting and divulging that, which they would not have come to open light, and which beside cannot be exprest in such modest terms, as are fit for the virginitie of pen & paper, and the white sheetes of their Child-bed. I must (as well as I can) defend my selfe from these imputations, and shew my care to keep both learning and modestie illibate, and inviolable … As for women (whom I am most afraid to offend) they must be content to have their infirmities detected, if they will have helpe for them, which I wish might not come to any eare or eye, but to those which they themselves would have acquainted therewith, and as well for their sakes, as mine owne satisfaction: I have endevoured to be as private and retired, in expressing al the passages in this kind as possibly I could.[20]

The translator thus declares himself appropriately concerned with bringing "to open light" the woman's body with all of the attendant discourse of shame and licentiousness: prostitution, divulging, violation. He is in concert with Guillemeau in this way, and he appears not to shy from promoting a sort of public-health message of his own that encourages women to benefit from this wisdom and swallow the inevitable shame: his prose is potentially life-saving. It is the arresting image of the virgin pen and the white sheets of childbed that remain with us, however. The productive pen must spill ink to express itself; no childbed sheets remain white for very long.

It is a document created for feminist critic Susan Gubar's discovery and delectation. Her groundbreaking work on women's creativity in nineteenth- and twentieth-century literature, most notably "'The Blank Page' and the Issues of Female Creativity," airs women's dirty laundry, as it were, and sees in both the stained sheets of the virgin's wedding bed and those that emerge shockingly pristine in the case of her lapsed sisters, a history of women—their bodies, their beds, and their books—as perpetually interwoven.

20 "Translator's Preface," in Guillemeau, *Child-birth*, p. 2.

> Because of the forms of self-expression available to women, artistic creation often feels like a violation, a belated reaction to male penetration rather than a possessing and controlling. Not an ejaculation of pleasure but a reaction to rending, the blood on the royal marriage sheets seems to imply that women's paint and ink are produced through a painful wounding, a literal influence of male authority. If artistic creativity is likened to biological creativity, the terror of inspiration for women is experienced quite literally as the terror of being entered, deflowered, possessed, taken, had, broken, ravished—all words which illustrate the pain of the passive self whose boundaries are being violated.[21]

Guillemeau and his translator are clearly dealing with the post-virginal woman's body, yet the ravishing of which Gubar writes is entirely consonant with the extreme trepidation with which male physicians approached the woman's body during birth. As for the translator's virgin pen–well, never has a case of phallic anxiety been more clearly construed. He as well fears the wrath of accusations for the improper use of his instrument. Alas, ink must be spilled in order to save women's lives, says he. Again, from Gubar:

> This model of the pen–penis writing on the virgin page participates in a long tradition identifying the author as a male who is primary and the female as his passive creation—a secondary object lacking autonomy, endowed with often contradictory meaning but denied intentionality. Clearly this tradition excludes woman from the creation of culture, even as it reifies her as an artifact within culture. It is therefore particularly problematic for those women who want to appropriate the pen by becoming writers. (Gubar 77)

Des Roches's experience is radically transformative of this notion of creativity as issuing from wounding or phallic penetration. The Athenian women greet Agnodice—the discoverer of their safety, the guardian of their health—with deep sensual, if not sexual, pleasure at the rediscovery of their learned selves, not far removed from the ejaculation of pleasure of which Gubar writes, yet utterly feminized: Catherine has, in effect, called upon Agnodice to lead her mother out of the misery of marriage and childbirth and shown light on a powerful, supportive, grateful, ecstatic community of women, free at last to touch and to tell.

[21] Susan Gubar, "'The Blank Page' and the Issues of Female Creativity" in Elizabeth Abel (ed.), *Writing and Sexual Difference* (Chicago, 1982), p. 86.

Chapter 4
Assimilation with a Vengeance: Maternity without Women in Male French Renaissance Lyric

> La société humaine est une anti-physis: elle ne subit pas passivement la présence de la nature, elle la reprend à son compte. Cette reprise n'est pas une opération intérieure et subjective: elle s'effectue objectivement dans la praxis.[1]
>
> [Human nature is an antiphysis—in a sense it is against nature; it does not passively submit to the presence of nature but rather takes over the control of nature on its own behalf. This arrogation is not an inward, subjective operation; it is accomplished objectively in practical action.]
>
> Simone de Beauvoir, *Le Deuxième sexe*

The poetry that inspired this chapter and the convening of sources as diverse as Pierre de Ronsard's odes and Simone de Beauvoir's *Second Sex* employs an image that unsettles the modern reader for its supposed unnaturalness. The concept of the breastfeeding male is arresting, even comical. Accustomed as we are to centuries of discourse on the natural processes of the nursing mother and to a small industry of scholarship by social historians on the subject, the suggestion of a lactating *father* in her stead elicits shock—a strange oxymoron that would appear to have a decidedly small field of investigation.[2] The evidence from humanists of sixteenth-century France, however, disproves this. The nursing father was a common *topos*, employed in a variety of literary settings to different effect. As such, a study of

---

1 Simone de Beauvoir, *Le Deuxième sexe 1* (Paris, 1949), p. 67. Translation: *The Second Sex*, H.M. Parshley (New York, 1974), p. 58. Unless otherwise indicated, translations are my own.

2 For illuminating treatment of this subject, see in particular Londa Schiebinger, *Nature's Body: Gender in the Making of Modern Science* (Boston, MA, 1993), specifically Chapter 2, "Why Mammals Are Called Mammals"; Mary Jacobus, "Incorruptible Milk: Breast-feeding and the French Revolution," in Sara Melzer and Leslie Rabine (eds), *Rebel Daughters: Women and the French Revolution* (Oxford, 1992), pp. 54–75; and Ruth Perry, "Colonizing the Breast: Sexuality and Maternity in Eighteenth-Century England," in John C. Fout (ed.), *Forbidden History: The State, Society and the Regulation of Sexuality in Modern Europe* (Chicago, 1992), pp. 107–37. Thomas Laqueur's pan-historical *Making Sex: Body and Gender from the Greeks to Freud* (Cambridge, MA, 1990) treats in depth the pre-Rousseauian discourse on the breast with several mentions of lactation in males.

this curious, albeit rather common literary convention whereby male authors appropriate such a highly female-defined function, offers important insight into prevailing attitudes toward gender and literature in early modern Europe. This chapter may prove the extremes of de Beauvoir's critique of historical materialism: human nature [la société humaine]—and in the context of this chapter I shall gender this male—does not heed a monolithic natural law. And indeed, men such as those quoted in this analysis do not stop short of coopting the woman's nursing body as their own, consuming her, becoming her, and transforming her—"[Il] la reprend à son compte!"—to promote and protect what remains a perpetually male literary universe.[3]

The project I undertake here discovers what a feminist critique of canonical male authors can tell us of how gender informs the praxis of men's writing of the Renaissance. Gender studies has revealed much about the literary strategies of early modern women writers and their inscription of gendered conventions and traditions in their works; with copious and diverse responses to de Beauvoir's legacy with regard to women writers now in mind, men's writing seems ripe for reappraisal. Ann R. Jones's groundbreaking article on this period, "Assimilation with a Difference," insightfully revealed the ways in which women writers strategized with male literary conventions to express a distinctly female condition. This work presents a converse operation with regard to their male counterparts: men as assimilators of women—their bodies, their domain, and their language—striving to construct a startlingly self-sufficient paradigm of literary sustenance and reproduction.[4] For the French Renaissance male poet, the maternal metaphor was an exceedingly attractive one for all it suggested in terms of rebirth and nourishment *vis-à-vis* a revered classical past. And so, just as Jones explored women's *bricolage* with male-defined convention and rhetoric, so does this chapter propose gendered readings of canonical male writers who masculinize maternity in order to empower their writing—coopting women and women's roles to further the cause of the French literary tradition, and, perhaps more importantly, their own quest for immortality. As they scavenge through Rome for edifying allusions and precedent, so do they pillage the female gender for all that it may afford their glorious project. Assimilation, as it were, with a vengeance.

Two examples of maternalized mentorship in the poetic works of Pierre de Ronsard present and pull into focus this peculiar dynamic: the first, an *elogia* to his teacher Jean Dorat; the second, a recasting of the same issues of praise and male nurturance with regard to a returning French statesman. Dorat, a renowned

---

[3] For a study of this question in the English Renaissance, see Katharine Eisaman Maus, "A Womb of His Own: Male Renaissance Poets in the Female Body," in James Grantham Turner (ed.), *Sexuality and Gender in Early Modern Europe: Institutions, Texts, Images* (Cambridge, 1993), pp. 266–88.

[4] Ann R. Jones, "Assimilation with a Difference: Renaissance Women Poets and Literary Influence," *Yale French Studies*, 62 (1981): pp. 135–53.

Renaissance Hellenist, known as the father of the group of poet luminaries named the Pléiade, and Ronsard, its most shining member, leave intriguing, literary traces of their mentor–disciple relationship, publicized most memorably in Ronsard's early poem "A Jan Dorat."[5] Ronsard's tremendous sense of privilege and personal mission combined with his consummate facility with the literary conventions of his day make him a fruitful primary subject for an analysis focused on issues of appropriation and masculine control.[6]

This chapter investigates principally the curious trope of the nursing father, but I begin by situating this maternalized male bond in the context of the appropriation of the birthing body itself, an image that was apparently dear to the discipleship of Ronsard and Dorat. In his "Hynne de Bacchus," Ronsard replays the myth of Dionysus (Bacchus), the typically effeminized god of wine and inspirer of liberating madness, with no small attention paid to his extraordinary birth. As we know from mythology, Bacchus is the issue of Zeus and Semele, a mortal. Pregnant with his child, Semele (through trickery from Zeus's jealous wife Hera) asks that the god reveal himself. Unable to withstand the blinding specter of this god of the gods, she perishes in the flames that attend his self-revelation. Zeus rescues the fetus from her womb and sews the prenatal Bacchus into his thigh to continue to gestate.[7] Ronsard explains:

> … ton pere te cacha
> Dedans sa cuisse ouverte, à fin que là tu prisses
> Ta forme et que tes mois comme au ventre accomplisses:
> Puis si tost que sa cuisse eut parfait justement
> Le terme où s'accomplist un vray enfantement,
> Il vint en Arabie, et comme une accouchée
> Qui sent avec douleur une longue trenchée,
> Rompit pour t'enfanter le bien-germeux lien
> De sa cuisse feconde au bord Sagarien. (vol. 2, 595)

---

5 Pierre de Ronsard, *Oeuvres complètes*, ed. Jean Céard, Daniel Ménager, and Michel Simonin (Paris, 1993), pp. 987–8. See also Appendix A for text and translation. All subsequent references are to this edition.

6 Ronsard's preface to the *Odes* of 1550, his first publication, conveys quite concisely his less than modest level of self-esteem: "Mais quand tu m'appelleras le premier auteur lirique François, et celui qui a guidé les autres au chemin de si honneste labeur, lors tu me rendras ce que tu me dois, et je m'efforcerai te faire apprendre qu'en vain je ne l'aurai receu." [Yet when you shall call me the first French lyric author, and he who has guided others in the path of such honest labor, then you shall render unto me that which you owe, and I shall work hard to prove to you that your praise was not unwarranted.] *Oeuvres complètes*, vol. 1, p. 994.

7 See Ovid's *Metamorphoses*, Book III, vv. 253–315, trans. Frank Justus Miller (Cambridge, MA, 1916 [reprinted 1984]), vol. III, pp. 143–7.

> [... your father hid you
> In his open thigh, so that you could grow
> And finish out your gestation as if in a womb:
> Then as soon as his thigh had perfected you,
> And brought you to term as with a real pregnancy
> He came to Arabia, like a woman in labor
> Who feels the pain of a long contraction,
> And broke open the germinating link to deliver you
> From his fecund thigh on the Arabian shores.]

This hymn was accorded rather extraordinary attention by Jean Dorat, who republished it in a special pamphlet edition (chez André Wechel, 1555) alongside his Latin translation.[8] The following treatment of the maternally characterized mentorship between Dorat and his star pupil will only invigorate the conception of men who seal their homosocial and academic bonds by means of the female body in parturition. There is much to suggest in what follows that this male gestation, surrounded as it is by the rhetoric "parfait," "vrai," "bien-germeux," and "fecond," is a felicitous appropriation of women's gift of birth that occurs clearly, conveniently, and perhaps necessarily, in their absence.

The Mentor's *feconde mammelle*

Ronsard's *éloge* of his (postpartum?) nursing mentor begins then:

> Puissai-je entonner un vers
> Qui raconte à l'univers
> Ton los porté sus son aile,
> Et combien je fu heureus
> Sucer le laict savoureus
> De ta feconde mammelle.
> Sur ma langue doucement
> Tu mis au commencement
> Je ne sçai quelles merveilles,
> Que vulgaires je randi,
> Et premier les épandi
> Dans les Françoises oreilles. (*Oeuvres*, vv. 1–12)
>
> [Could I but intone a verse
> That would tell the world
> Your glory carried on its wing,
> And how fortunate I was

[8] See *Oeuvres complètes*, vol. 2, n. 2, p. 1473.

> To suckle the savory milk
> Of your fertile breast!
> Upon my tongue sweetly
> Did you place at first
> Indescribable marvels
> That I rendered into French,
> The first to pour them
> Into French ears]

Not surprisingly for those familiar with Ronsard, this ode penned ostensibly to honor his beloved teacher Dorat ends up speaking mainly about himself. This is a common phenomenon throughout his works, most notably in the *Amours*, where his praise-weary lovers—Cassandre, Marie, and Hélène—stand in as models for his personal literary agenda. Ronsard's famous depiction of Hélène's lament, "Ronsard me célébrait, du temps que j'étais belle" [Ronsard celebrated me in the time of my youthful beauty], is typical of this self-interested strategy. "Puissai-*je*" [Could *I*], he begins, and rarely refocuses attention away from his own subjectivity. Dorat becomes a pretext for talking about Ronsard's greatness. The back and forth between Ronsard and Dorat in this poem is a structuring mechanism indeed: puissai-*je*—*ton* los, *je* fu heureus—*ta* mammelle, *ma* langue—*tu* mis, and so on; but the emphasis is clearly on the success of Ronsard. The poem ends, after all, not with direct praise of Dorat, as in "you are so knowledgeable and wonderful," but instead with "Voi m'en ci le temoignage" [See in me the witness of this greatness], literally, "Look at *me*!" The practice of coopting the subjects of his work and employing them for personal gain—be they lovers, mothers, and/or mentors—is deeply relevant to Ronsard's poetics and emblematic of the same impulse one finds in his contemporaries. A quick summary of the remainder of the poem should make clear Ronsard's intentions.

It is the duty of a student, he explains in the next two stanzas, to pay homage to one's teacher—emphasizing again "le miel de *ma voix*" [the sweetness (honey) of *my voice*] and *his* (Ronsard's) laureled head. At the midpoint in stanza five, Ronsard returns to the imagery of the opening in slightly modified terms. Again, he begins "si *j'ai* du bruit" [if *I* am famous] then concedes it is because of his preceptor's fine tutoring—a teacher who *found* him *thirsting* [Tout alteré me treuva] and gave him drink [m'abreuva]—"de l'une et l'autre fontaine" [from both fountains (sources)]. This reference to the two fountains of the Muses, Castalia and Hippocrene, harkens back to the breasts from his opening, as well as, metaphorically, to Greek and Latin, the languages of Antiquity so key to Ronsard's apprenticeship in letters. Stanza six reiterates the name of the *mother* as mentor to the apprentice who, while young, may please the common public [les bandes rurales] yet who when fully formed, targets the more discerning, more educated, and, as in "mains liberales," more remunerative royal court. The Ronsard–Dorat relationship is then recast in the Olympian context—Dorat as generous minister or Phoebus-Apollo to Ronsard's grateful, adoring muse, which leads to a final, self-interested description of how contented and proud Dorat must feel to have suckled a child such as he, Ronsard, witness to Dorat's greatness, which now firmly belongs to them both. So concludes this poem written ostensibly to praise the mentor, and working simultaneously to immortalize the apprentice as well.

Some 20 years later, Ronsard offered another version of the nursing male, this time describing Monseigneur le Connétable (the uncle of his addressee, the Cardinal de Chatillon) as wet nurse to an adoring, thirsting nation. What appeared in the poem to Jean Dorat as supporting a literary agenda is reworked here into a political message. Monseigneur le Connétable returns to his countrymen as a bountiful mother whose breast will nourish and warm his hungering charges. The thirst for knowledge that is slaked in his earlier poem is here conflated with a thirst for leadership and moral authority:[9]

> … Comme un petit enfant que sa nourrice avoit
> Allaité longuement pleure s'il ne la voit,
> De ses petites mains au berceau se tourmente,
> En soupirant l'appelle, et toujours se lamente
> D'une voix enfantine, et ne veut s'éjouir
> Jusqu'à tant qu'il la voie ou qu'il la puisse ouïr;
> …
> Elle en ses bras l'échauffe, et depuis le matin
> Soigneuse jusqu'au soir le pend à son tétin:
> Ainsi toute la France à l'heureuse venue
> De ton oncle captif joyeuse est devenue. (vv. 1–6; 9–12)
>
> [Like a baby whose wet nurse had
> Suckled him for so long and cries if he can't see her,
> His little arms flailing vainly in torment
> Sadly crying out to her, lamenting inconsolably
> In his newborn call, bereft and unhappy
> Until he can see or hear her;
> …
> She warms him in her arms, and from morning
> Until night, carefully holds him to her nipple:
> Such is France's joy at the most happy
> Return of your captive uncle.]

France, here depicted as the hungry, male child, awaits the return of his wet nurse, again a man, who will suckle his adoring countrymen back to health and contentedness. This, from a poet whose epic verse, however unsuccessfully, attempted to rival the bellicose strains of Virgil's *Aenied.*[10] The mother soon

[9] Pierre de Ronsard, "Le Retour d'Anne de Mont-Morency Connestable de France à Odet de Colligny, Cardinal de Chastillon," in *Oeuvres complètes*, vol. 2, pp. 818–19.

[10] See Ronsard's *La Franciade* (1572), *Oeuvres complètes*, pp. 1011–159.

disappears, however. Men, even warriors, now suckle their sons. One sees here how the image of the nursing male remained a powerful metaphor for Ronsard across genres, and within the various paradigms of desire, consumption, and satiety that these literary configurations entailed. In a literary milieu obsessed with the celebration and rebirth of classical origins for the purpose of legitimizing and "nourishing" the French vernacular tradition, Ronsard strives in a variety of ways to transform and implicate the male spirit and body as part of the imaginings of creation and sustenance of national leadership and literary prowess. In this masculinist poetics, Ronsard appropriates for men the role of bountiful mother who may dispense and imbibe at will to disciples, peers, and countrymen with an abundance of maternal warmth and fecundity exacted from their idealized female others. As subsequent examples demonstrate, Ronsard's strategy of appropriation was not unique: male glorification and edification via maternal discourse was common to a variety of contemporaneous writers. Having presented one poet's particular versions of this theme, however, some preliminary suggestions as to the provenance and general currency of the maternal male are in order. Investigation of the logic of such seemingly unusual poetic rhetoric is illuminated by an analysis of both *literary* convention and precedent and other more *literal*, scientific suppositions of the early modern period. What emerges is a set of conveniently crafted assumptions about gender and (re)production that persistently favor male dominance and control—a preponderant iconography of men vested with women's maternal functions, supported and sustained in both poetic and anatomic constructs.

Just as Ronsard's *lovers* served his self-interest as *porte-paroles* of his changing literary agenda, so is the *mother* coopted in quite similar ways by the opportunistic lyricist. The poet's engagement with Petrarchan poetic convention easily repermutates from one female role to another. Ronsard's relation to female lovers as well as maternal figures betrays a more generalized appropriation of the female persona in order to better totalize his literary control. Philippa Berry's study of male Petrarchan poets and their relation to the female lover resonates well with practices of the same group of writers with regard to mothers, and responds quite appropriately to the specific case of Ronsard's poem:

> This figure [of the beloved] was usually little more than an instrument in an elaborate game of *masculine* "speculation" and self-determination, for the philosophical enterprise common to both Petrarchism and Renaissance Neoplatonism used woman as a "speculum" or mirror of masculine narcissism. The hypothesis that a chaste woman could serve as a bridge between the material world and an invisible spiritual dimension enabled Petrarchan poet and Neoplatonic philosopher to elaborate *a new concept of masculine wholeness and self-sufficiency* through or across her idealized figure. By this means, they

> affirmed Renaissance man's conviction that he could achieve a godlike control, not just over his own nature, but over his environment as well.[11]

By focusing on another female role that is exploited and appropriated by male writers, this poetry suggests that men were not constrained entirely within the realm of the chaste and idealized body of the Platonic, female lover in order to achieve "masculine wholeness and self-sufficiency," but worked "through or across"—and indeed *as* or *within*—the maternal body in order to further this godlike control over their own nature and environment: shades of de Beauvoir come back to mind—"elle ne subit pas passivement la présence de la nature, elle la reprend à son compte" [it does not passively submit to the presence of nature but rather takes control of nature on its own behalf]. By expanding the paradigm that Berry uses in her analysis, we see in Ronsard and his contemporaries a vision of the male poet as ever more controlling, their agenda perhaps only more insidious and predatory. The desire for the female lover becomes conflated with the desire for creative control, an ideal more logically centered in the female breast and womb than heart.

Berry's exploration of masculinist control of women and nature as witnessed in their manipulation of Petrarchan conventions appears only more keenly relevant to Ronsard and Dorat when paired with theories of male homosociality. The discussion of the female lover and her conflicted role as essential to male creativity yet ultimately irrelevant or incommodious is the subject of Eve Sedgwick's pioneering treatment of Shakespeare.[12] Sedgwick illuminates this recurring image of male poets bonding over the ubiquitous female object of desire and consumption in a way that is only further expanded by examining men as observers and consumers of mothers. Sedgwick defines the process of female inclusion and eventual effacement within the male literary world as programmatic, even normative. As with Berry, Sedgwick's claims are for a male/female erotic love construct—"the compulsory routing of homosocial desire through heterosexual love more or less as a matter of course" (Sedgwick 160). The refiguring of their paradigms with respect to mothers as opposed to lovers disturbs little the economy of their desire for immortality. Just as in Shakespeare's sonnets, where the poet and his rival joust and bond over the Dark Lady (as in Sedgwick's Girardian configuration), so do Ronsard and Dorat raise the specter of woman, only to absorb her (embody her) and continue on unfettered. Women become the site for male union and then, de- or re-materialize in their poetic works as masculinized mothers.

Interestingly, in terms of homosocial theory, Ronsard plays out the paradigm in a way that is at once more expansive and more efficient than the triangular configuration originally suggested. In Ronsard's poem, we know Dorat to be

---

[11] Philippa Berry, *Of Chastity and Power: Elizabethan Literature and the Unmarried Queen* (London, 1989), p. 2 (my emphasis).

[12] Eve Kosofsky Sedgwick, *Between Men: English Literature and Male Homosocial Desire* (New York, 1985).

at once a collaborator or mentor to Ronsard as well as, in this instance, a muse figure. Dorat's reputation as a crafter and teacher of poetic verse is collapsed into his inspirational role, here expressed through a depiction of him as mother. He thus performs double duty in the male–female–male triad, a feat accomplished by Ronsard's supernatural suggestion of his mentor as endowed with maternal capacities. Ronsard thus configures and controls both his muse *and* his modes of production, imbibing and embodying roles traditionally reserved for women. Woman is most certainly still implicated in Dorat and Ronsard's poetic enterprise; she is, however, entirely absorbed. The praise that in most other Petrarchan situations belonged at least ostensibly to the lover is here clearly that of the men.

Nurturing the Single-Sex View

The question of men working *within* the maternal body to assume literary control of their poetic subjects is only furthered in contemporaneous literature on human anatomy. The last several decades of theorizing on early modern conceptions of sex and gender have brought to light a vision of male and female conflation that suggests that what Ronsard imagines might have been grounded in physiological reality. In the Renaissance world view, Dorat was already more maternal than more modern critics might give him credit for. Writers on the body from as early as Galen and forward to Ambroise Paré explained sex and gender under the assumption of anatomical sameness, the woman's genitalia being left "undescended." Thomas Laqueur's analysis of prevailing conceptions converges on the view of an "oxymoronic one-sex body."

> It is a … body whose fluids—blood, semen, milk, and the various excrements—are fungible in that they turn into one another and whose processes—digestion and generation, menstruation and other bleeding—are not so easily distinguished or so easily assignable to one sex or another … This "one flesh," the construction of a single-sexed body with its different versions attributed to at least two genders, was framed in antiquity to valorize the extraordinary cultural assertion of patriarchy, of the father, in the face of the more sensorily evident claim of the mother.[13]

Within this paradigm, then, with regard to sex, the process of appropriation had already been suggested to men. Notions of what the male body was capable of and how it functioned allow for a somewhat less perplexed reaction to Ronsard's depiction of his nursing mentor. Men had been "making their milk and drinking it too" since antiquity, and for very good reasons it would appear. The "extraordinary cultural assertion of patriarchy" expressed by Laqueur conveniently and convincingly mirrors the "godlike control of nature" proposed in Berry's literary

[13] Thomas Laqueur, *Making Sex*, pp. 19–20.

paradigm. Thus, Ronsard expresses literarily what Laqueur sees as a powerful cultural impulse to control and define a male hegemonic code. Medical, scientific discourse set in place a view to man's naturally androgynous physical being that finds expression in these literary imaginings. Male breastfeeders speak to a condition that is less "appropriation" then, than expression, or perhaps exploitation, of an already integrated body capable of male and female functions.

What is clearly important is that this quasi-hermaphroditic conception of the body for men is worked consistently to their advantage. Men do not become weakened or effeminized by dint of their embodiment of both male and female properties; on the contrary, they become ever more male, ever more perfect. Here, medical and literary imaginings of the Renaissance diverge in interesting ways. Ambroise Paré, the royal surgeon to the French court, includes a chapter in his 1573 work, *Des Monstres et des prodiges* [Of Monsters and Marvels], entitled "Histoires Memorables de Certaines Femmes Qui Sont Dégénérées en Hommes" [Memorable Stories about Women Who Have Degenerated into Men]. Paré relates indeed quite memorable and fantastic stories from the past of women who, when their natural processes of heat exhalation are blocked, may well, with a sudden jolt, experience an expulsion of their previously internalized genitalia. The story made famous by Montaigne of Marie Germain, whose sex changed as she jumped a stream while chasing her pigs, is the author's final dramatic example. Paré concludes his physiological explanation with the following observation:

> Or, comme telle metamorphose a lieu en Nature par les raisons et exemples alleguees, aussi nous ne trouvons jamais en histoire veritable que d'homme aucun soit devenu femme, pour-ce que nature tend tousjours à ce qui est le plus parfaict, et non au contraire faire que ce qui est parfaict devienne imparfaict.[14]

> [So, just as this metamorphosis takes place in Nature for the reasons and in the examples here alleged, we never find, thus, a reputable story of any man become woman, for Nature evolves always to that which is more perfect and not, on the contrary, making that which is perfect imperfect.]

And so, though the single-sex theory of anatomy implies a fungibility of fluids and a certain indeterminacy of sexual identity, Paré is quick and sure to offer a misogynist truism that points to inevitable transformation toward that which is perfect and male and away from the cold, troubled humors of woman. What Ronsard imagines in his poem, however, is not so much that Dorat abandons his perfect sex, but rather enjoys a literary transvestism of sorts that affords him the control of body and of word, a "praxis," as de Beauvoir would have it, that does not "passively submit" to Nature's laws. He indeed subverts them. The masculinist voice is only more empowered for the surplus of imagined maternal capacities.

[14] Ambroise Paré, *Des Monstres et prodiges*, ed. Jean Céard (Geneva, 1971), p. 30.

Dorat may don for him all that the mothering male may afford him and shed it at will, certain of his status rejoined to the fraternity of poets he has spawned.

Fraternal Bonding at the Breast

Given this contextualization of Ronsard's poetics of maternal appropriation, there remains an array of similar literary texts where the recurrent image of men as mothers further illuminates this masculinist agenda. The "père nourrisseur" [nourishing father] resurfaces within many of Ronsard's peers' writings, both secular and religious. The following examples reveal a variety of ways in which other male writers engaged the maternal figure on their behalf, further expanding our appreciation of the popularity of this image for men across decades, literary genres, and political agendas. These poets' inscription of the maternal male also plays into and transforms many of the poetic conventions of their male literary tradition—all of them converging on a common view to male glorification and a concomitant, gradual effacement of the female body which they put into temporary poetic service.

Ronsard's fellow Pléiade member Rémy Belleau, in his *Amours et nouveaux eschanges des pierres précieuses* [Love Poems and Exchanges on Precious Stones] of 1576, speaks of paternal nourishment, transforming a common literary convention in which traditionally female and or maternal imagery is thoroughly masculinized. Belleau writes in geological metaphor of the rivers, characterized as masculine, that nourish and form the material galactite (perhaps the mineral known as talc):

> Le Nil et l'Achelois, grands fleuves de la terre,
> Dans leur sein limmoneux nourrissent ceste pierre,
> De couleur blanchissante et de mesme saveur
> Que le lait, des enfans le pere nourrisseur. (vv. 77–80)[15]
>
> [The Nile and the Achelois, great rivers of the Earth
> In their silty breast nourish this stone
> Of whitish hue and of the same taste
> As milk, [this stone] the nourishing father of children.]

Belleau participates here in a common literary trope for writers of his century, that of poetic allusion to regional rivers that flow through writers' birthplaces and that are honored for having inspired and, in a metaphysical sense, produced them. The Loire and Loir garnered much praise from Ronsard and Du Bellay for having birthed, nourished, and inspired their vastly productive poetic careers. Similarly,

[15] Rémy Belleau in *Poètes du XVIe siècle*, ed. Albert-Marie Schmidt (Paris, 1953), p. 659.

the confluence of the Rhône and Saône rivers in Lyon is worked into the strains of many of that city's writers, most consistently by Maurice Scève, who depicts the felicitous joining of two rivers into one as symbolic of both male–female romantic union and the resultant fertility of the Lyonnais environs, which produces and inspires its renowned poets. Scève declares in *dizain* XVII: "Plutôt seront Rhône et Saône déjoints/Que d'avec toi mon coeur se désassemble" [Sooner would the Rhone and Saone disunite/Than would my heart from yours break away].[16] That Belleau revises this *topos* in a way that does away with the female influence is telling, and quite compatible with similarly male-defined paradigms penned by his peers. Mother Nature cedes to "père nourisseur." And, as if to underscore this miraculous, male *coup de force*, the mineral produced by this fecund father river—the "père/pierre nourrisseur"—is said by Belleau to assist in the production of milk when applied to the breast.[17]

Just as the father's breast might signal goodness and nourishment, so might it convey the opposite: the source of corruption. Another Pléiade member, Pontus de Tyard, in his "Du Socratique," Ode III, also masculinizes the maternal breast in his depiction of male nourishment and influence when speaking of Epicurus, this time portraying the counter-example, the "père nourrisseur" gone bad:

> Luy, comme les inhumains,
> Qui feirent au Ciel la guerre
> Pour l'egaler à la terre,
> Sentit les divines mains
> Assommer les discours vains
> Dedans sa poitrine infecte,
> Qu'encor depuis ont teté
> Les nourrissons de la secte
> Qui souille la Deïté. (vv. 10–18)[18]

---

[16] Maurice Scève, *Délie*, ed. Françoise Charpentier (Paris, 1984), p. 61.

[17] Belleau writes (Schmidt, *Poètes du XVIe siècle*, vv. 41–4, p. 658):

> Or cest pierre donc qu'on appelle Laicteuse
> Fait enfler le tetin de l'humeur gracieuse,
> Qui arrose en maillot la lévre des enfans,
> Et qui les nourrisant fait accroistre leurs ans.
>
> [So this stone that is called "Laicteuse" (milky)
> Fills the teat with that grace-giving fluid,
> That moistens the swaddled infants lips
> And while nourishing them, increases their years.]

[18] Pontus de Tyard, "Ode III: Due Socratique," from the *Livre des Vers Lyriques* (1573), in Schmidt, *Poètes du XVIe siècle*, p. 380.

[He, like those barbarians
Who make war with Heaven
To reduce it to earthly dimension
Felt the divine hands
Break asunder the vain discourse
Within his filthy breast
From whence have suckled
The disciples of this sect
That sullies God.]

While the pure, male, nursing breast can pour forth the milk of human kindness and true compassion, so might its polluted twin—the "poitrine infecte"—pass on evil and degeneration. While Ronsard and Belleau insist on the positively idealized qualities of the mothering breast and exploit it to express a miraculously masculinized version of fecundity and nutriment, Tyard plays on the more physical and therefore dangerous suppositions of women's corporeal nature: bodies as changeable, polluted, and vulnerable to nefarious forces of corruption. As Juan Luis Vives admonishes in his contemporaneous *Education of a Christian Woman*: "I pray thee, understand thine own goodness maid, … shut up both body and mind, and seal them with those seals that none can open."[19] Vives's anxiety regarding young women's habit of attending tournaments of arms gets right to the point:

> But a young woman cannot easily be of chaste mind if her thoughts are occupied with the sword and sinewy muscles and virile strength. What room do these thoughts leave for chastity, which is defenseless, unwarlike, and weak? A woman who contemplates these things drinks poison into her breast, of which such interest and such words are symptoms.[20]

Commensurate with commonly held anatomical notions of the period, women's imagination was seen as capable of corrupting her child *in utero* as well as her milk; here, it has been transferred onto the male poet. Tyard puts into play the notions of pollution and degeneracy that both influence and issue from the mother and then translates this nefarious threat onto a *male* nursing figure, here depicted as contaminated rather than glorified by association with the maternal body. The maternal breast could therefore be appropriated in completely opposite ways depending upon the poet's agenda, an arbitrariness comparable to the fate of poetic lovers. If Ronsard's Marie could be praised as the hallmark of a new "style bas,"

---

[19] Juan Luis Vives, *Instruction of a Christian Woman*, cited in Joan Larsen Klein (ed.), *Daughters, Wives and Widows: Writings by Men about Women and Marriage* (Chicago, 1992), p. 104.

[20] Juan Luis Vives, *The Education of a Christian Woman: A Sixteenth-Century Manual*, ed. and trans. Charles Fantazzi (Chicago, 2000), p. 73. This editor works from a different edition of Vives's work, of which there were many in the sixteenth century.

so could she later be cast off as too simple, a vestige of a previous poetic agenda. Likewise, in these poetic appropriations of the maternal role, the nursing mother may stand in for divine bounty or contaminated vessel of sin and corruption at the whim of the scribe. Women in these male lyric poets' universe, whether lovers or mothers, are malleable and ultimately disposable.

The authors examined thus far hail from the literary fraternity of Pléiade poets whose maternal fantasies exhibit a common rhetoric of infinite control over the content and the destiny of their writing. While these men had individual (and at times rival) agendas, their poetics have been seen as functioning within a homosocial dialectic that edifies male production and self-sustainment. These male poets assume the natural processes of women, exploiting and explaining them in ways which praise (Ronsard and Belleau) or caution (Tyard) regarding the powerful effects of male mothers. In the remaining examples, the analysis moves within and beyond the Pléiade sphere and explores how the use of the maternal metaphor transformed larger, commonly held literary and iconographic depictions of poetic creation, here again invoking the maternal and gendering it male. Readings of Rabelais, Aubigné, and Du Bellay push our analysis from breast to womb, furthering the vision of the totalizing control of women's bodies enacted by this savvy generation of male writers.

One of the better known examples of maternalized mentorship among male humanists is that of François Rabelais's letter to Bernard Salignac (1532); the true addressee was Erasmus. Having referred to Erasmus as "Pater mi Humanissime," Rabelais continues:

> Patrem te dixi, matrem etiam dicerem, si per indulgentiam mihi id tuam liceret. Quod enim utero gerentibus usui uenire quotidie experimur, ut quos nunquam uiderunt fœtus alant ab aërisque ambientis incommodis tueantur … qui me tibi de facie ignotum, nomine etiam ignobilem sic educasti, sic castissimis *diuinae tuae doctrinae uberibus usque aluisti*, ut quidquid sum et ualeo, tibi id uni acceptum [21]
>
> [I have called you "father," I might say even "mother," if you would indulge me in this sentiment. In fact, pregnant women nourish a fetus that they have never seen and protect it from the perils of the outside world … you have never seen my face, even my name was unknown to you and yet you educated me, *you have not ceased from nourishing me with the irreproachable milk of your holy knowledge*; what I am, what I am worth, I owe entirely to you.]

Again, as with Ronsard and Dorat, we see the praise of a mentor figure who employs the maternal metaphor in order to describe the apprenticeship and growth of the learner. In some translations, the "diuinae tuae doctrinae uberibus" is rendered

[21] François Rabelais, *Oeuvres complètes*, ed. Mireille Huchon (Paris, 1994) pp. 998–9 (my emphasis).

from Rabelais's Latin "uberibus" as, logically, "mamelles" or teats. The English translation of *uber* connotes richness, fruitfulness, fertility and alternately breast, teat, udder, or dug.

Several influences appear to be at work in Rabelais's epistle. Rabelais is in dialogue here with his mentor in ways which bespeak an intertextual relationship as well as a common view to Renaissance poets' conception of indebtedness to classical precedent. The concept of pairing the nursing breast with the dispensing of knowledge, whether divine or humanist, held great currency in the sixteenth-century literary milieu. Childrearing manuals and scholarly ruminations concerning the imbibing of milk and of knowledge are consistently wont to link the two activities as one. Conduct books, such as Juan Luis Vives's previously cited *Education of a Christian Woman*, admonish women to breastfeed their own children and cultivate their minds simultaneously as the two phenomena are interdependent.[22] Erasmus himself was similarly convinced and replicates much of this text (and its classical precedent, which is most surely Plutarch's "On the Training of Children") in his own work "On the Education of Children," suggesting the conflation of men, nursing, and learning presented more tacitly in his predecessors. Having concluded his remarks on nurses, Erasmus turns to the timely selection of a tutor. Contrary to popular thought, which advises indulging children in their carefree youth, he claims:

> Instead, you should straightaway begin to search for a man of good character and respectable learning to whose care you may safely entrust your son to receive the proper nourishment for his mind and to imbibe, as it were, with the milk that he suckles, the nectar of education.[23]

If it was suggested before in the case of Ronsard and Dorat that feminization precedes appropriation, it appears that re-masculinization of the mentor and disciple is an equally important part of this dialectic. Further iconographical evidence may offer some insights.

For the learned Renaissance audience, this maternalization of the mentor bespeaks as well an attachment to the highly recognizable theme of *innutrition* or nourishment which characterized the Pléiade poets' relationship to knowledge and inspiration in general, and to their Latin and Greek ancestors in specific. Joachim Du Bellay, another Pléiade member, describes this most clearly in his *Deffence et illustration de la langue Françoyse* of 1535, wherein he speaks of emulating the Romans whom he describes as:

---

22 In addition to the previously cited editions of Vives, see also the *Livre de l'institution de la femme chrestienne*, trans. Pierre de Changy (1542), reprinted with preface and glossary by A. Delboulle (Le Havre, 1891); and Foster Watson, *Vives and the Renascence Education of Women* (New York, 1912) for extensive reproduction and translation of the text.

23 Desiderius Erasmus, *De Pueris Instituendis,* in *Collected Works of Erasmus*, ed. J. K. Sowards (Toronto, 1985), p. 299.

> immitant les meilleurs aucteurs Grecz, se transformant en eux, les devorant, & apres les avoir bien digerez, les convertissant en sang et nourriture, chacun selon son naturel[24]
>
> [imitating the best of the Greek authors, transforming oneself into them, devouring them, and after having well digested them, converting them into blood and food, each one according to their own style.]

Images of appropriation and oral sustenance seem keenly applicable. The process of transforming, digesting, and being reborn is entirely suggestive of the phenomenon of maternalization and subsequent appropriation—seen here as devouring—that these authors are enacting. Not only do these writers become and devour their literary ancestors, however; this same transformation and consumption pertains to women. Feeding off women, just as Du Bellay would have it described of the Greeks, the Renaissance writer empowers his poetry with all that his opportunistic pen can glean. The comment "chacun selon son naturel" only further emphasizes the convenience and adaptability of this poetic strategy. Thus, the works of Du Bellay and his male contemporaries, however conflicted in their relation to the past, express highly similar impulses to biologize, and more specifically to maternalize, the process of the creation of a viable, French literary agenda. Their theses are predicated on the notion of maternal language, of naturalness of expression passed on through evolving *generations* of writers indebted to but distinct from a Greek and Latin past which cannot fully respond to their emerging sense of national identity.

Thomas Sébillet, in his *Art Poétique*, maps out this generational ancestry most exhaustively and the absence of female participation or inclusion is revealing. In a passage redolent of Old Testament rhetoric, he intones the "begats" of literary precedent:

> De la (Apollo, Arion, Amphion, Orphée) Homère, de la Hesiode, de la Pindare … de la le plaisant Plaute trouvarent nom et faveur entre les Romains: et apres euz Virgile, Ovide, Horace…les Italiens, retenans encor quelque vestige de ce florissant empire par le moien d'un Danthe et d'un Petrarque. [E]t les François … Jan de Meun, et Jan le Marie, divine de race, et digne de roial entretien.[25]
>
> [From Apollo and Orpheus came Homer … whence came Hesiod, then Pindare … from whence Plautus who found fame and favor among the Romans: after whom Virgil, Ovid, Horace … then the Italians who retained some vestiges of this flourishing empire by way of Dante and Petrarch … [A]nd the French …

---

[24] Joachim Du Bellay, *La Deffence et illustration de la langue Françoyse*, ed. Henri Chamard (Paris, 1970), p. 42.

[25] Thomas Sébillet, *Art Poétique*, ed. Félix Gaiffe and Francis Goyet (Paris, 1988), pp. 13–14.

> Jean de Meun and Jean Lemaire de Belges, of divine lineage, and worthy of royal patronage.]

The mothers in this process have vanished. Sébillet's genealogy is a male poetic conceit that suggests female absorption into what remains an entirely masculine descent. If Ronsard and his peers suggest the means by which this is possible, Sébillet simply expresses the ends: male writers, male tradition, male reproduction.

The Lupine Breast

With Sébillet and Ronsard particularly in mind, Joachim Du Bellay's famous sonnet IX from *Les Regrets* provides a telling commentary on conceptions of gender and literary ancestry evoked by writers of his century:

> France, mere des arts, des armes, et des loix,
> Tu m'as nourry long temps du laict de ta mamelle:
> Ores, comme un aigneau qui sa nourrice appelle,
> Je remplis de ton nom les antres et les bois.
>
> Si tu m'as pour enfant advoué quelquefois,
> Que ne me respons-tu maintenant, o cruelle?
> France, France, respons à ma triste querelle:
> Mais nul, sinon Echo, ne respond à ma voix.
>
> [France, mother of arts, mother of arms and laws,
> You gave me suck from your abundant breast:
> Now like a lamb crying for what is lost
> I fill the rocks and forests with my call.
>
> If at one time you admitted I was yours,
> Why are you silent now, why are you cruel?
> France, oh France, answer me mercifully!
> But the echo only brings back my own words.][26]

Du Bellay depicts himself here as a helpless lamb/child, wandering the Roman countryside in search of the breast of his mother, his mother's milk, the *langue maternelle* which can sustain him, and which, not inconsequentially, he has fought to define and defend. If "France, mother of arts" places woman at the center of this maternal personification, the evidence gleaned from contemporaneous accounts suggests the transparency of this claim. Ronsard has maternalized Jean Dorat,

[26] Joachim Du Bellay, *Les Regrets*, ed. Françoise Joukovsky (Paris, 1971), pp. 64–5. Translation: C.H. Sisson (Manchester, 1984), pp. 26–7.

the father of Renaissance court poetry, and claimed Monseigneur le Connétable as "nourrice" to his country; Sébillet's genealogy clearly marks the effacement of female involvement; and Tyard even suggests that maternalized males are as capable of corruption as women themselves. Indeed, Du Bellay's regrets and sense of abandonment during his sojourn in Italy, where his poems are penned, harken back not so much to this idealized Mother France as to a group of male poets whose celebrity and favor with the court threaten to outstrip him.

The implication of a male presence and tradition in control behind the facade of the mother country is more explicit later in Du Bellay's poem where he evokes lupine imagery and a mythological account of parenthood and nurturance quite fitting to this discussion: "Entre les loups cruels j'erre parmy la plaine" [I am left to wander among hungry wolves]. The poet/lamenter depicts himself as orphaned, wandering about the countryside, in search of sustenance, in the presence of wolves. Du Bellay begs comparison with the Roman sucklers *par excellence*, Romulus and Remus, a reprise of Rabelais's "uber"—the breasts, dugs, or teats. And images return of Ronsard, found thirsting by a Dorat *qua* Faustulus, the shepherd who discovered the abandoned twins, suckled by a she-wolf. Du Bellay's sonnet is an elegant depiction of his conflicted relationship with two mothers, two "sources": France and Rome. France, the good-wolf/mother is absent and Du Bellay wanders Rome, tormented, agonizing as he does textually throughout the *Regrets* and *Deffence* about his relationship to the Roman legacy, alluded to as the roving, carnivorous "bad-wolf."[27]

This nursing wolf challenges our conceptions of maternity in much the same way as Ronsard's depiction of Dorat. Suckling at the breast of an aging male mentor or under a wild she-wolf seems at first glance a similarly unnatural, inappropriate activity. If it is Dorat's gender that unsettles the reader, it is the wolf's animality, an animality accentuated by a visual code that is clearly, again, masculine. The most famous icon of the Roman lore is the Capitoline Wolf, a bronze visited like a shrine during the Renaissance by legions of enthralled humanists, drinking (nursing?) at the source, as it were, of their reborn world of letters. Bernard Andreae's popular

[27] Du Bellay's sonnet "Une Louve je vy," from his collection *Songe* (1558), complements the version in the *Regrets* with a more literal rendering of the story (the French gender distinction expressed by *loup/louve* is decidedly less clumsy than the English translation). Schmidt, *Poètes du XVIe siècle*, vv. 41–4, p. 658.

> Une Louve je vy sous l'antre d'un rocher
> Allaictant deux bessons: Je vis à sa mamelle
> Mignardement joüer ceste couple jumelle,
> Et d'un col allongé la Louve les lecher …
>
> [A She-Wolf I spied in a rocky cave
> Nursing two twins: I saw at her breast
> This twin couple gently playing
> As the She-Wolf stretched back her neck and licked them …]

description of the statue from *The Art of Rome* expresses most efficiently the gender flux at work in the poetic renderings of this image:

> The forelegs are rigidly blocked in place, as if the animal had stopped short. The back legs with their muscular shanks are supplely relaxed but ready, at an instant's need, to swing the body around to face an aggressor from any direction. The wedge of the body culminates in the half-open muzzle with its bared fangs. The dilated nostrils sniff the air for an enemy scent, tense veins shoot across the muzzle, the folds above the eyes are sharp … Wide open, erect, the ears emphasize the impression of alertness. The tightly superimposed curls of the mane are like flames, and they continue in a crest along the back all the way to the tail (a later restoration), circling the entire forepart in a tight girdle just behind the shoulders. The flanks of the lean but powerful beast are sucked in, its ribs protrude …[28]

As this description rather unsubtly suggests, the image of the Roman she-wolf is highly masculinized, with its female features quite consciously reconstrued—the dugs themselves, given the "sucked in flanks" and protruding ribs, appear more phallic than maternal. If Du Bellay, Ronsard, and their contemporaries are searching for a male model of maternal sustenance, this icon would appear to serve the purpose well. The strangeness of the twins suckling at this phallic, bestial mother resonates with and neatly prepares the image of the young male poet suckling at the breast of his mentor. Natural, maternal functions are conveniently revised. The iconography circulating at the time suggested a fluidity of gender, leaving it up to Renaissance male writers to incorporate and transform its power and meaning.

Male Self-Sufficiency Perfected

The opening to Agrippa d'Aubigné's *Tragiques* provides appropriate material for a conclusion to this analysis in that it pushes the concept of male appropriation of the maternal body to its most powerful end: the male poet who produces his own (textual) progeny and is then suckled by this child-become-mother. From "L'Auteur à son Livre":

> Va Livre, tu n'es que trop beau
> Pour estre né dans le tombeau
> Duquel mon exil te delivre;
> Seul pour nous deux je veux perir:
> Commence, mon enfant, à vivre
> Quand ton pere s'en va mourir.

[28] Bernard Andreae, *The Art of Rome*, trans. Robert Erich Wolf (New York, 1977), p. 37.

> Encores vivrai-je par toi,
> Mon fils, comme tu vis par moi;
> Puis il faut, comme la nourrice
> Et fille du Romain grison,
> Que tu allaicte & tu cherisse
> Ton pere, en exil, en prison. (vv. 1–12)[29]
>
> [Go, my Book, you are too beautiful
> To have been born in this tomb
> Into which my exile has delivered you;
> Alone, I shall perish for us both:
> Begin, my child, to live
> When your father goes to die.
> I shall live again through you,
> My son, as you were given life by me;
> Thus you must, like the wet nurse
> And daughter of the Roman prisoner,
> Suckle me & cherish
> Your father, in exile, in prison.]

Aubigné, engaging another relevant literary *topos* popular among his literary peers, addresses his book as his child that he has created and that he hopes will outlast him and continue to give testimony to his worthiness as a writer.[30] Aubigné illustrates this convention with an allusion to the legend of the Roman girl who visits her famished father in prison and breastfeeds him across the bars to keep him from starving. Aubigné thoroughly masculinizes the story to speak of his own, tightly controlled universe of literary production. *La nourrice* becomes *mon fils*, a son begat, in effect, by literary parthenogenesis. Furthermore, as in Ronsard's regendering in "La Nourrice," the original legend cited by Garnier and Plattard in their edition of *Les Tragiques* tells the story of a *mother*, not a father, who is imprisoned and subsequently nursed by her daughter.[31] In Aubigné's version then, once again, the women vanish. There is no woman's body left in his story and we are left with the recurring image of men suckling men.[32] With Aubigné,

---

[29] Agrippa d'Aubigné, *Les Tragiques*, ed. A. Garnier and J. Plattard (Paris, 1990), p. 17.

[30] See as well Ronsard's "A Son Livre" ("Mon fils, si tu savais ce qu'on dira de toi …"), in *Oeuvres complètes*, pp.167–72.

[31] "L'origine de cette légende est une anecdote de Valère-Maxime (*Factorum ac dictorum memorabilium libri*, au livre V, chap. IV, 7), chez qui d'ailleurs *c'est une mère, et non un père*, qui est ainsi allaitée par sa fille." *Les Tragiques*, p. 17, note (my emphasis).

[32] For an extended discussion of Aubigné's relation to the maternal as it evolved over his entire career, see Kathleen P. Long's "Motherhood and Martyrdom in the Poetry of Théodore Agrippa d'Aubigné," *Neophilologus*, 76/2 (1992): pp. 198–211. According to

the maternalized homosocial triad that was streamlined in the case of Ronsard and Dorat is entirely collapsed into one utterly self-sufficient and self-sustaining paradigm. Aubigné is the birth *father* of his own son, who subsequently enjoys the same powers of supernatural gender fluidity that allow him to suckle his starving father in return. How much simpler, one cannot help observing, for Aubigné to have suggested the book as "daughter"; simpler, yet unwelcome in a genealogy of female erasure and exclusion and male, poetic control.

If the image of men nursing their literary progeny is more rarely invoked, the idea of birthing them was certainly not: men birthing books were commonplace. Indeed, the thesis about breastfeeding males might easily be seen as a subset of a much broader phenomenon of men as child*bearers*. The "children of the spirit" privileged by Renaissance readers of Plato's *Symposium* were commonly cited and it is that source that certainly informs the scenarios of suckling mentors that I have discussed within this study. Perhaps the most famous Renaissance practitioner of literary male birthing was Michel de Montaigne, whose "De l'affection des peres aux enfans" [On the Affection of Fathers for their Children] offers pertinent and often-quoted observations that show the extent to which women—their bodies, their functions (both physical and social)—can be appropriated and effaced within a male literary agenda:

> (C)ar ce que nous engendrons par l'ame, les enfantemens de nostre esprit … sont produicts par une plus noble partie que la corporelle, et sont plus nostres; nous sommes pere et mere ensemble en cette generation.
>
> [For what we engender by the soul, the children of our mind … are produced by a nobler part than the body and are more our own; we are father and mother both in this generation.]
>
> …
>
> Et je ne sçay si je n'aimerois pas mieux beaucoup en avoir produict ung, parfaictement bien formé, de l'acointance des muses, que de l'acointance de ma femme.
>
> [And I do not know whether I would not like much better to have produced one perfectly formed child by intercourse with the muses than by intercourse with my wife.][33]

Long, Aubigné's maternity works not only in the service of his own poetic immortality, but as representative of a larger agenda of Protestant salvation and sacrifice: "He [Aubigné] sees the ultimate role of the poet as a maternal rejection of violence through literary creation … It is the poet's maternal role to give new life out of the fire to these martyrs, to restore their voices in the hope of putting an end to sacrifice" (209–10).

[33] Michel de Montaigne, *Essais*, Livre 2, ed. Alexandre Micha (Paris, 1969), pp. 71, 73. Translation: *The Complete Essays of Montaigne*, Donald M. Frame (Stanford, 1976),

Aubigné simply extends the metaphor that much further, allowing this nobler enterprise to continue to nourish its own without the messy interventions of "l'acointance de [l]a femme." The "nous" and "notre" [we and our] are clearly the rhetoric of a male literary bond that indicates a perpetually masculine privilege enthralled with maternal functions to the extent to which they can be transformed and owned by men.

Ronsard and his contemporaries' relationship to the maternal was identical to the very process of imitation and apprenticeship they sought to express. Just as Homer, Ovid, Petrarch, and others are "devoured, digested, and converted," to borrow Joachim Du Bellay's terminology, just as the wisdom of Dorat is sucked from his breast and made manifest in the "body" of writing penned by Ronsard, so is the mother consumed and transformed by these still unquestionably male appropriators. As these diverse variations of the mothering male have shown, the plundering of maternity was the not-uncommon *modus operandi* of this generation of writers bound for glory. Controlling nature through women's bodies on their own behalf, as de Beauvoir's rhetoric suggests at the beginning of this chapter, male writers of the French Renaissance birthed a self-sustaining literary tradition unencumbered by natural mothers.

***

A brief epilogue is provided here to conclude a chapter that has dwelt so relentlessly on female exclusion and silence in a male literary tradition. I return again to the example of Louise Boursier, midwife to the French court in the early seventeenth century, and friend and follower (with her husband) of Ambroise Paré, who authored several works on her experiences in the profession of assisting real women in real births (see Chapter 2). Her prefatorial writing in the work *Observations diverses sur la stérilité, perte de fruits, fécondité, accouchements, et maladies des femmes et enfants nouveau-nés* [*Some observations on sterility, miscarriage, fecundity, births and illnesses of women and newborns*] provides a welcome antidote to the masculinist verse that plays at maternity yet willfully avoids its "acquaintance." She begins her "Au Lecteur":

> Ami lecteur, cet enfant de mon esprit … ne s'étale point à tes yeux pour se faire admirer en la vanité du langage. Il te dit pour une de ses maximes véritables, qu'il n'a point le fil d'une Ariane pour te conduire avec un plaisir doucement trompeur, parmi les contours d'un labyrinthe de paroles. Aussi ne lui ai-je donné pour tout fard que la vérité, pour raison que l'expérience, et pour témoin tout notre sexe, qui ressentant en soi-même ce que j'en écris ne démentira jamais ma plume.[34]

pp. 291, 293.

[34] Louise Boursier, *Observations diverses sur la stérilité, perte de fruits, fécondité, accouchements, et maladies des femmes et enfants nouveau-nés* (1609), ed. Françoise Olive

> [Friendly reader, this child of my spirit … is not displayed before you to be admired for the vanity of its language. It holds as a truth that there is no Ariadne's thread that can guide you with sweet deception among the twists and turns of a labyrinth of words. So have I given it no mask but the truth, no reasoning but experience and as witness all those of our sex, who, able to feel within themselves that which I write about will never repudiate my writing.]

Louise Boursier's words might indeed be the opening of the complementary chapter to this study. The "notre sexe" suddenly and clearly refocuses the attention on women whose maternal potential or actual experience presents a radical revisioning of what this child of the spirit entails. Claiming to be suspicious of rhetorical tricks or literary imaginings (such as those, we might conjecture, that would make mothers out of men), Boursier pens prose that is literally life-giving and sustaining. Boursier comes out of the dark shadows of male imagination and dismissal and bears witness to her own experience in poetry, in anecdotal accounts of her birthing experiences and remedies, and in cautionary, epistolary prose to her own daughter. Her "observations" are a link to a tradition of women's writing born of women's bodies, a tradition thoroughly elided in the Renaissance, male poetic agenda.

(Paris, 1992), p. 31.

Chapter 5

Unstable Bodies: Birthing Monstrosities in Early Modern France

> [F]inally, and always, people construct gender as well as the social systems that are grounded in gender-based concepts … Accepting genital ambiguity as a natural option would require that physicians also acknowledge that genital ambiguity is "corrected" not because it is threatening to the infant's life but because it is threatening to the infant's culture.[1]
>
> Suzanne Kessler

> The body—what we eat, how we dress, the daily rituals through which we attend to the body—is a medium of culture. The body, as anthropologist Mary Douglas has argued, is a powerful symbolic form, a surface on which the central rules, hierarchies, and even metaphysical commitments of a culture are inscribed and thus reinforced through the concrete language of the body.[2]
>
> Susan Bordo

This chapter is about what men, or bodies perceived to be male, can and cannot be, can and cannot do according to certain arbiters of gender in early modern France. Having explored in the previous chapter the ways in which male writers appropriated the maternal *literarily*—exploiting the *topoi* of birth and nursing as metaphors for their literary (re)production—I turn now to accounts of men's assumption of these roles more *literally*. Within the popular literature of this period one finds accounts of men, or male-looking persons, who transgressed the perceived limitations of their sex and gave birth. The most common condition that gives rise to the question of male maternity, and the one that I investigate here, is that of hermaphrodism: persons of ambiguous genital configuration whose primary and secondary sex characteristics advertise a gender seemingly at odds with the capacity to reproduce. The stories of mutable, inscrutable, and ambiguous bodies evoked an intense fascination and anxiety, an uneasiness that looked often to the realm of a vagrant imagination, immorality, or satanic intervention as its cause.

I contribute to the work on hermaphrodism of this period by treating selected graphic and literary sources from contemporaneous works and by engaging more

---

1 Suzanne Kessler, "The Medical Construction of Gender: Case Management of Intersexed Infants," *Signs: Journal of Women in Culture and Society*, 16 (1990): p. 25.

2 Susan Bordo, "The Body and the Reproduction of Femininity," in Katie Conboy, Nadia Medina, and Sarah Stanbury (eds), *Writing on the Body: Female Embodiment and Feminist Theory* (New York, 1997), p. 90.

current discourse on intersexuality that may serve to enliven the discussion of this locus of persistent social apprehension. This fascination and anxiety clearly endures, as Kessler's admonition from the epigraph suggests ("finally, and always"): modern-day regulations of who is male and who is female, of what is male and what is female, and of why these remain our only two options collapse into enduring, rigid categorization. Two early twenty-first-century gender conundrums relay this well: the case of Caster Semenya, a South African runner whose victory at the 2009 World Athletics Championship in the women's 800-meter event was thrown under intense scrutiny based on characterizations of her sex; and Thomas Beatie, who in that same summer gave birth to his second child. As *The New York Times* announced, "He's Pregnant. You're Speechless."[3] We may debate long and productively over one- and two-sexed conceptions of the body at play at the beginning of the seventeenth century and how they inform more or less capacious views of sex and gender (see Chapter 4); but in the end, the hegemony of "normative" gender assignment has remained largely binary, reductive, and often punitive. I follow Kessler in discovering the ways in which hermaphrodites signaled not only their own personal calamity, but also that of their culture.

In addition, I take my cues from Judith Butler who, in *Undoing Gender*, speaks to the intersexual and gender regulation as instructive both for the ways in which sexual indeterminacy is troublesome for those who live at "the limits of intelligibility" as well as for her honest and compassionate defense of the rights to desire and love in ways that refute the arbiters of one's gender. The consequences of sexual ambiguity in a society that demands coherent gender as a presupposition of humanness are fraught and, as in the case that she treats in the chapter "Doing Justice to Someone," sometimes fatal:[4]

> When we ask, what are the conditions of intelligibility by which the human emerges, by which the human is recognized, by which some subject becomes the subject of human love, we are asking about conditions of intelligibility composed of norms, of practices, that have become presuppositional, without which we cannot think the human at all. (57)

I apply Butler's interrogations without apology to an era far removed from the contemporary cases causing such controversy today. Narratives of sexual aberration from the early modern era do much to nourish and elucidate the sense of the "regular" and the "regulatable" (57) that endure. Butler's privileging of narrative and agency is instructive and deeply humanizing to the ancestors of the Caster Semenyas and the Thomas Beaties, whose interstitial lives of unrecognizablity,

---

[3] See Jeré Longman, "South African Runner's Sex-Verification Result Won't Be Public," *The New York Times*, 19 November 2009, and Guy Trebay, "He's Pregnant. You're Speechless," *The New York Times*, 22 June 2008 (regarding Thomas Beatie's first pregnancy).

[4] Judith Butler, *Undoing Gender* (New York, 2004), pp. 57–74.

inscrutability, and intense social and juridical regulation are well served by our attention to the past; whose political motivations, though recast, are not so very different from our own.

My primary text for introducing the ambient discourse surrounding hermaphrodism (if not initially allied with birthing *per se*) is Thomas Artus's fantastical *L'Isle des hermaphrodites* of 1605, which presents the question of gender transgression by parodying the person and the court of Henri III as an utterly unstable and risible locus of debauchery. Henri III was, certainly, a man though copious reports of his predilection for women's finery (politically motivated as they were) might betray a certain playfulness with gender. He was not a hermaphrodite. To use the accusation of hermaphrodism as the cornerstone of this parody is to press into service a robust and persistent anxiety around gender in this period, a fear of sexual ambiguity closely woven into the political, social, religious, and medical discourse of his time.[5] I link Thomas Artus's text with two pertinent and popular works published on either side of the *Isle*: *Histoires prodigieuses*, by Pierre Boaistuau (1560), augmented in later editions by Claude Tesserant (1567) and François de Belleforest (1571, 1598); and *Des Hermaphrodits …* (1612) by Jacques Duval. Both texts are invested in a narrative about men's sexual ambiguity that entertains and instructs their readership in ways that resonate with *L'Isle des hermaphrodites*. I investigate Artus's premise and consider the stakes of hermaphrodism as it might pertain to corrupted, curdled masculinity, and put into question, as Bordo encourages, the cultural commitments inscribed in a variety of bodily images and accounts from the period. My exploration unfolds into a discussion of unconventional birthing bodies, beginning with Artus's satirized hermaphrodism, a narrative that impugns its subject precisely because one of the hermaphrodite's primal transgressions is to throw into question the most radical obligation attached to the bi-gendered *Zeitgeist*, that of the clear separation of male and female for the very purposes of reproduction and regeneration. To treat birthing bodies and hermaphrodism in the same space is to invite trouble. I propose to engage this anxiety and illuminate examples that can both feed and allay this social apprehension.

Before embarking on the voyage, as it were, to the island of hermaphrodites, it is perhaps best to make the distinction between the androgynous and the hermaphroditic, as both of these terms are invoked in the examples to follow. Gary

---

[5] From the small industry of scholarship dedicated to the question of propaganda and debauchery as pertaining to Henri III and his *mignons*, see Joseph Cady's "The 'Masculine Love' of the 'Princes of Sodom' 'Practising the Art of Ganymede' at Henri III's Court: The Homosexuality of Henri III and His Mignons in Pierre de L'Estoiles' *Mémoires-Journaux*," in Jacqueline Murray and Konrad Eisenbichler (eds), *Desire and Discipline: Sex and Sexuality in the Premodern West* (Toronto, 1996), pp. 123–54; and Katherine B. Crawford, "Love, Sodomy, and Scandal: Controlling the Sexual Reputation of Henry III," *Journal of the History of Sexuality*, 12 (2003): pp. 513–42.

Ferguson's investigation of the androgyne with respect to women of precisely this time period and literary milieu delineates this as follows:

> The origins of the hermaphrodite, going back to the story of Hermaphroditus and Salmacis in the fourth book of the *Metamorphoses*, are quite different from those of the androgyne, since Ovid's story is one not of doubleness and completion, but of emasculation and diminishment. Salmacis's name disappears as she joins with Hermaphroditus, her effect on the latter being only to weaken and effeminise him. If the androgyne generally had positive connotations, susceptible to idealising allegory, the hermaphrodite, on the contrary, tended to be associated with real human beings.[6]

The messiness of "real human beings," perceived to be at odds with or toying with their sex and gender, is persistently nefarious. Todd Reeser concurs with this, declaring the accusation of hermaphrodism as pejorative because of its violence to masculinity specifically. Speaking directly of the Artus text, he claims:

> In the *Isle*, which explicitly evokes the Ovidian model to explain the origin of the hermaphroditic race … it is clear that feminine gendered traits are repeatedly superimposed onto an at least largely male body and that a fallen masculinity is more the issue than sexual or gender fluidity *per se*.[7]

The inscription of hermaphoditism onto the body is necessarily deleterious, as it works against the Galenic model (reiterated by Ambroise Paré and others in the sixteenth century) that evinces the ever-perfecting human body as evolving from female to male.[8] To parody men as hermaphrodites is to suggest the incomprehensible and radically unnatural specter of women's genitals as mapped onto men, a reversal of biological and medical wisdom that simply could not be. It is in the context of such heteronormative imperatives that the power of the unstable island kingdom claims currency.[9]

---

[6] Gary Ferguson, *Queer (Re)Readings in the French Renaissance: Homosexuality, Gender, Culture* (Aldershot, 2008), p. 266.

[7] Todd Reeser, *Moderating Masculinity in Early Modern Culture* (Chapel Hill, 2006), p. 242.

[8] For an excellent presentation of the pertinent texts, see Kathleen P. Long's first chapter in *Hermaphrodites in Renaissance Europe* (Aldershot, 2006), pp. 29–47.

[9] One of the radical distinctions to be made between the early modern period and the cases that inform Judith Butler's theory in *Undoing Gender* (and which would deserve much more lengthy treatment elsewhere) is the much higher prevalence of male to female, versus female to male sexual reassignments. Butler decries the medical practitioners and regulators of such operations whose wisdom declares "the ease with which a female body can be surgically constructed, as if femininity was always little more or less than a surgical construction, an elimination, a cutting away" (Butler 64).

Unstable Island Life

Following a long and adventure-filled voyage of escape and discovery, the narrator of Artus's *L'Isle des hermaphrodites* decides to return to Europe, newly pacified after the tumultuous events of the latter half of the sixteenth century. A ship sets sail for Lisbon from an unnamed land across the ocean and, in the tradition of true adventure tales, within very short order the weather starts getting rough, the ship is tossed, and eventually sets ground on the shore of an uncharted desert isle. The passengers, grateful to be alive, disembark. To their surprise:

> nous veismes que la terre sur laquelle nous marchions estoit toute flotante, et qu'elle erroit vagabonde sur ce grand Ocean sans aucune stabilité.[10]
>
> [we saw that the ground upon which we were walking was all afloat and was drifting aimlessly over this great ocean with no stability whatsoever.]

The travelers quickly realize that they have traded one floating community for another and that this one is defined, naturally and culturally, by instability. The skipper heads off in one direction and the narrator toward a luxurious palace not far off:

> [D]e là nous entrasmes dans une grande court de laquelle *le pavement estoit si luisant et si glissant qu'à peine s'y pouvoit on tenir*. Toutesfois l'envie de passer plus outre nous feit aller tous chancelans au grand escalier … (58, my emphasis)
>
> [From there, we entered into a grand courtyard *whose pavement was so bright and shiny that we could barely remain upright*. All the same, our desire to explore further encouraged us shakily on toward the grand staircase.]

The wide-eyed visitors stumble freely about, discovering to their perpetual amazement an island in the thrall of sexual indeterminacy. The palace is abuzz with the activities of an important inhabitant's morning regimen: "The Hermaphrodite" is rising and the frantic minions rush about with a fantastic assortment of accoutrements to assist in a daily, torturous ritual. This privileged hermaphrodite, referred to as "he," is preened, primped, and squeezed into a portrait of the most extravagant, effeminate delicacy imaginable. Once the hair is curled and powdered, the limbs kneaded and stretched, the waist cinched, and the feet hammered into the tiniest of shoes, he rises:

[10] Thomas Artus, *L'Isle des hermaphrodites* (1605), ed. Claude-Gilbert Dubois (Geneva, 1996), p. 56. All translations are my own unless otherwise noted.

> [L]ors commença à se remuer de luy-mesme, car jusques alors il n'avoit eu mouvement que par l'ayde d'autruy; mais *il bransloit tellement le corps, la teste et les jambes que je croyois à tous propos qu'il deust tomber de son long*. J'avois opinion que cela leur arrivoit, à cause de l'instabilité de l'isle, mais j'y appris depuis que c'est à cause qu'ils trouvent ceste façon là plus belle que pas une autre. (68, my emphasis)

> [And then he began stirring on his own, for up until then he hadn't made any unassisted movement; *but his torso, head, and legs were flailing about such that I thought that at any moment he'd fall flat on his face*. I was thinking that this was due to the island's instability, but I later learned that it was because they find this way of walking more beautiful than any other.]

The trope of instability in Artus's tale is pervasive and all-consuming, the bizarre comportment of the inhabitants perfectly mirrored in their surroundings.[11] Reeser has cogently analyzed this text's radical instability as illustrative of a lack of moderation with regard to sanctioned male deportment—what he would term "nonmoderate" behavior—and draws the connection between the tyrannical and the effeminate in important ways. His discussion is couched in terms of the official injunction against female rule and the much scrutinized influence of the forceful Catherine de Médicis over her son. Henri's lack of adherence to virile norms is the sign of aberration that fuels the tension in Artus's text. As Reeser states, "This anxiety is often mediated through discussions of tyranny in which the effeminate ruler risks breaking Salic Law by acting like a woman. Thus, as in the Greek tradition, acting tyrannical is similar to acting effeminate because both

---

[11] This comportment is parodied similarly in Agrippa d'Aubigné's "Princes" from *Les Tragiques* (1616), the classically scornful contemporaneous critique of the Valois court. The performance of the effeminized monarch is altogether commensurate with the bobbing and weaving of these court *mignons*. Aubigné and Artus operate from within the same dystopic paradigm of transgressing and transvesting transexual regents. Agrippa d'Aubigné, *Les Tragiques*, ed. A. Garnier and J. Plattard (Paris, 1990), p. 92:

> Il reste que le corps comme l'accoustrement
> Soit aux loix de la cour: marcher mignonnement,
> Trainer les pieds, mener les bras, hocher la teste,
> Pour bransler à propos d'un pennache la creste.

> [And so the body like an accoutrement
> Conforms to the laws of the court: prancing preciously,
> Dragging the feet, waving the arms, bobbing the head,
> To set dancing about the feathers on their hats.]

imply losing control over the self" (Reeser 239).[12] Implied in Henri's purported abdication of virile deportment as well is the refusal of the duty of producing an heir, a charge not unfamiliar or unfitting for Henri III, who had no issue with Louise de Lorraine. In a society that did not accept the rule of women, Henri's satirized effeminacy maps personal predilections with regard to gender transgression onto hereditary catastrophe. Again, Aubigné, whose enraged verse spews a toxic mix of accusations—pederasty, whoring, sterility, infanticide, incest, and Italian depravity—encapsulates the horrors of their perverse, transgendered rule well:

> Mais mal-heureux celui qui vit esclave infame
> Sous une femme hommace & sous un homme femme! (Aubigné 53)
>
> [Unhappy is he who lives hideously enslaved
> Under a manly woman and under a womanly man!]

Returning to *L'Isle* and its satirical critique of the debauched performance of gender, we find that the narrator eschews any description of himself or his fellow travelers, a narrative strategy whose effect is to invite us into his world with great immediacy, discovering along with and through him this strange island in meticulous, sensory detail. In fact, all bodies in *L'Isle des hermaphrodites* remain extremely elusive, perhaps in order not to lose hold of the critique of the monarch who is, after all, male. As Kathleen P. Long duly underscores in her treatment of the work:

> Throughout his satirical novel about the court of Henri de Valois, Artus seems obsessed with the cultural signs of gender—clothing, gesture, language, public behavior—rather than bodily marks of sex or reproductive questions … This outward appearance in turn creates the hermaphroditic identity, rather than echoing some inherent quality.[13]

One might conclude from Artus's meticulous attention to sartorial detail that the clothes make the hermaphrodite. Henri III is consciously corrupting his male body; his preening and mincing is an abomination that he is visiting upon himself, a self-

[12] As for the trope of the floating island, Reeser appears to want to have it several ways. He first states, "The instability of the island … symbolizes not so much the instabilities of gender but those of masculinity" (243), and then later, "In fact, the floating island strikingly parallels Aristotle's description of the 'movement' in the womb, and the island itself to the 'embryo' or the biological 'mother' of the hermaphrodites, held responsible for their gender instabilities" (250). I am comfortable with Reeser's capacious, if somewhat unstable analysis in this regard.

[13] Kathleen P. Long, *Hermaphrodites in Renaissance Europe*, p. 216. For connections of Artus's text to various depictions of the court of Henri III by contemporaneous detractors, see pp. 202–3.

imposed degradation of his God-given sex and gender. We as readers are witness to this abomination and our reading is a constant act of decoding and discernment of the "hermaphrodite's" immoral behavior.

This interpretive act is suggested to us most clearly not far into the story. The narrator has been touring about from room to room and comes across yet another hermaphrodite. "He" has been dressed and made up much in the manner of the first example and click-clacks away on his bejeweled velour mules behind a tapestry. The narrator wishes to follow, but, uncharacteristically, is turned away: this inner sanctum is reserved for a most restricted entourage:

> [J]e les vouloy suivre, car il me sembloit que tout estoit permis, et que l'entrée ne me devoit point estre deffendue … mais on me dict qu'ils tenoient icy leurs conseils plus secrets, et traictoient là de leurs privez affaires. De sorte que personne n'y avoit d'accez, que les plus familiers. (73)

> [I wanted to follow them, for it seemed to me that all was permitted and that my entrance should not be denied … but they told me that this was where they held their most secret council and dealt with their private affairs. Accordingly, none but the most intimate acquaintances had access.]

He is made to wait outside in an antechamber where, to pass the time, he contemplates the scenes woven into the tapestry dividing him from the secret activities. Several tell the story of Heliogabalus, a notoriously debauched Roman emperor whose attempts to transform himself from male to female end quite unsuccessfully:

> En une autre piece, je voyois ce mesme homme estendu tout nud sus une table, et plusieurs à l'entour de luy qui avoient diverses sortes de ferremens, et faisoient tout ce qui leur estoit possible pour le faire devenir femme; mais à ce que j'en pouvois juger par la suitte de l'histoire il demeuroit du genre neutre. (73)

> [In another tableau, I saw this same man laid out entirely naked on a table with several attendants around him bearing various and sundry iron tools doing all that was possible to make him into a woman; but from what I could gather from the rest of the story, he remained neuter.]

This tapestry might serve as a cautionary tale were the narrator to find himself enamored of this strange new world; the example of Heliogabalus as inscribed on a partition between the narrator and the unseen, unknown world of trans/intersexual intimacies is also, however, a fruitful starting place for a discussion of unstable bodies. Like the narrator, like any curious visitor in a strangely constructed world, we want to see what is "behind the curtain." To get there, I propose my own "decryption" of related works that treat the phenomenon of mutating male bodies and that, not inconsequentially, are often embedded in the discourse on hermaphrodites. My discussion focuses on a variety of aberrant male bodies—monstrous, indeterminate, even maternal—that stood as symbols for what society could and would not tolerate. The profoundly unstable setting of *L'Isle des hermaphrodites* is a gateway into a discussion of transgressive men's bodies—and of bodies of men's writing—writ large.

Portraits of Corruption

I begin by returning to the story of Heliogabalus, the narrator's waiting room reading material, as it were. His reaction to the tapestry is at once naïve and matter of fact. The inherently disturbing vision of the naked subject being operated on by several attendants wielding various metal instruments for the purpose of changing his sex is undercut by the brevity of the description and the admission of the viewer's uncertainty: "from what I gather, the operation wasn't successful." The contemporary reader of Artus, however, may well have gathered more information which would have informed his reception of the story, namely, Pierre Boaistuau's wildly popular *Histoires prodigieuses les plus memorables …*, published for the first time in 1560 and re-edited in compilations numerous times thereafter. This compendium of monstrosities from a variety of ancient and early modern sources includes in the final book (as augmented by Claude Tesserant in 1567), "Histoire d'un homme avec des cheveux de femme" [Story of a man with women's hair]. The chapter contains, strangely, no direct mention of a man of such physical qualities and uses the occasion instead to tell the story of Heliogabalus in all its gory detail wherein the whoring, cross-dressing, sodomizing, self-mutilating protagonist is, along with his mother, decapitated, dragged through town, and sunk to the bottom of the Tibris river:

> La teste fut couppee à l'un & à l'autre, leurs corps despouillez nuds furent premierement trainez par toute la ville ignominieusement … on iecta celuy du fils en une cloaque qui estoit l'esgoust de toutes les ordures de la ville … on le traina iusques au Tibre, dedans lequel on le iecta apres luy avoir attaché quelques poids pesans, afin que son corps ne flottast sur l'eau, & qu'il ne fut ensevely.[14]
>
> [Both of their heads were cut off, [and] their bodies, stripped naked, were dragged humiliatingly through the city … they threw the son's body in a cesspool that served as the gutter for all the city's garbage … and dragged him through it to the Tibris, into which they threw him after having attached heavy weights to him so that he wouldn't float and be found for burial.]

[14] Pierre Boaistuau, Claude Tesserant, and François de Belleforest, *Histoires prodigieuses les plus mémorable qui ayent esté observées depuis la nativité de Jésus-Christ, jusques à nostre siècle: extraictes de plusiers fameux autheurs grecz et latins, sacrez et prophanes* (Paris, 1598), pp. 419–20.

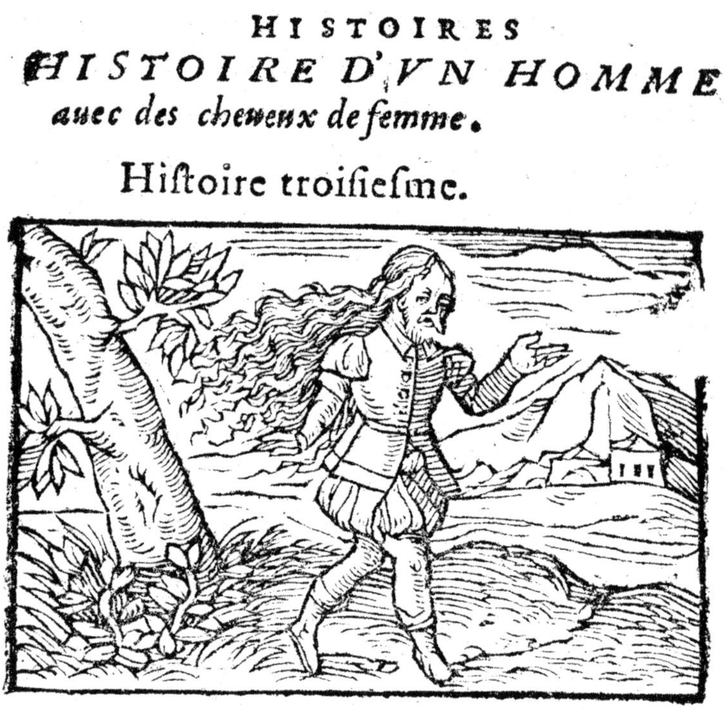
HISTOIRES

HISTOIRE D'VN HOMME avec des cheveux de femme.

Hiſtoire troiſieſme.

Figure 5.1 Man with the hair of a woman, Pierre Boaistuau, *Histoires prodigieuses* (1567), [25228.18.9.2]. Courtesy of Houghton Library, Harvard University.

A cautionary tale indeed. Tesserant's dramatic text is preceded, however, by an intriguing woodcut of the strangely coiffed man (Figure 5.1).[15] The man in question trips along merrily in a natural setting, long hair billowing out dramatically from the right side of his head. He has just passed a tree, and a large mountain looms in the background with the hint of a city or town sketched up against it. While he is clearly moving from left to right with haste, the engraver is at pains to depict a frontal view so as to demonstrate the bifurcated nature of the subject: he sports seemingly two outfits at once, the right side of the doublet parting slightly to reveal the more voluminous fabric of the breeches of the other. His hands are raised in a gesture of self-display, palms open, up and facing the viewer. The man appears to be fleeing the town in the distance and, by contrast with the large tree that mimics his gestures, utterly *un*natural—a perverse folly of courtly fashion. If it is not meant to be a literal depiction of Heliogabalus, it certainly

[15] For a brief discussion of the woodcuts in Boaistuau's work and their dissemination in other publications of the period, see Ruth Luborsky, "The Pictorial Image of the Jew in Elizabethan Secular Books," *Shakespeare Quarterly*, 46/4 (1995): pp. 449–53.

brings forth the central vice in question: a confusing composite of a man on the run from a society that will eventually track him down and do him in.

The seeming disconnect between the title, woodcut, and text in this chapter serves to heighten the transgressive power of this body: as will be shown below, the *Histoires prodigieuses* did not shy from disturbing images—a more literal depiction, say, of the debauched and mutilated protagonist. The drama resides, rather, in the somewhat frantic performance of effeminacy that the man with women's hair enacts. As with Artus's hermaphrodites, the dramatic coiffure, the hand, the elaborately tailored outfit, in sum, the artifice of transgressed masculinity is what is at stake. In contrast with the host of monstrous beings contained within the text—a man with several heads, children with a plethora of limbs, interspecial monstrous composites—long, flowing locks seem pretty tame fare. Women's hair is the synecdoche of the monstrous business of gender transgression. In the early modern, pre-DNA world view, this mane testifies more to the sin of straying outside one's gender than about a regrettable, biological anomaly (as are most of the other examples). The woodcut—in its own way a tapestry guarding the entrance to the tale of Heliogabalus—warns quite efficiently of the peril to come, a peril manufactured by his own hand.

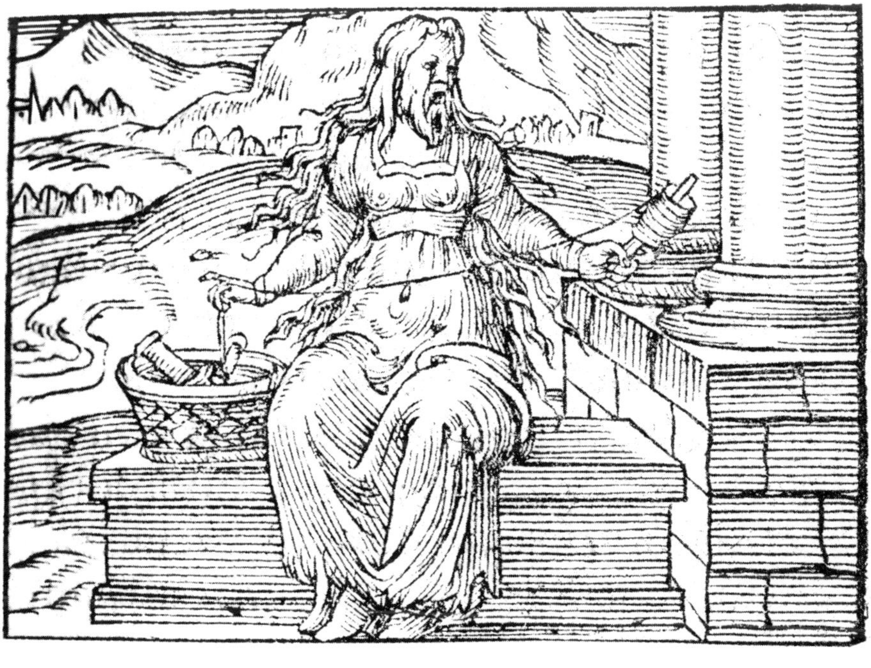

Figure 5.2 Man with the hair of a woman, Pierre Boaistuau, *Histoires prodigieuses* (1597–8). Courtesy of Dartmouth College Library [GR825.B63.1597 v. 1].

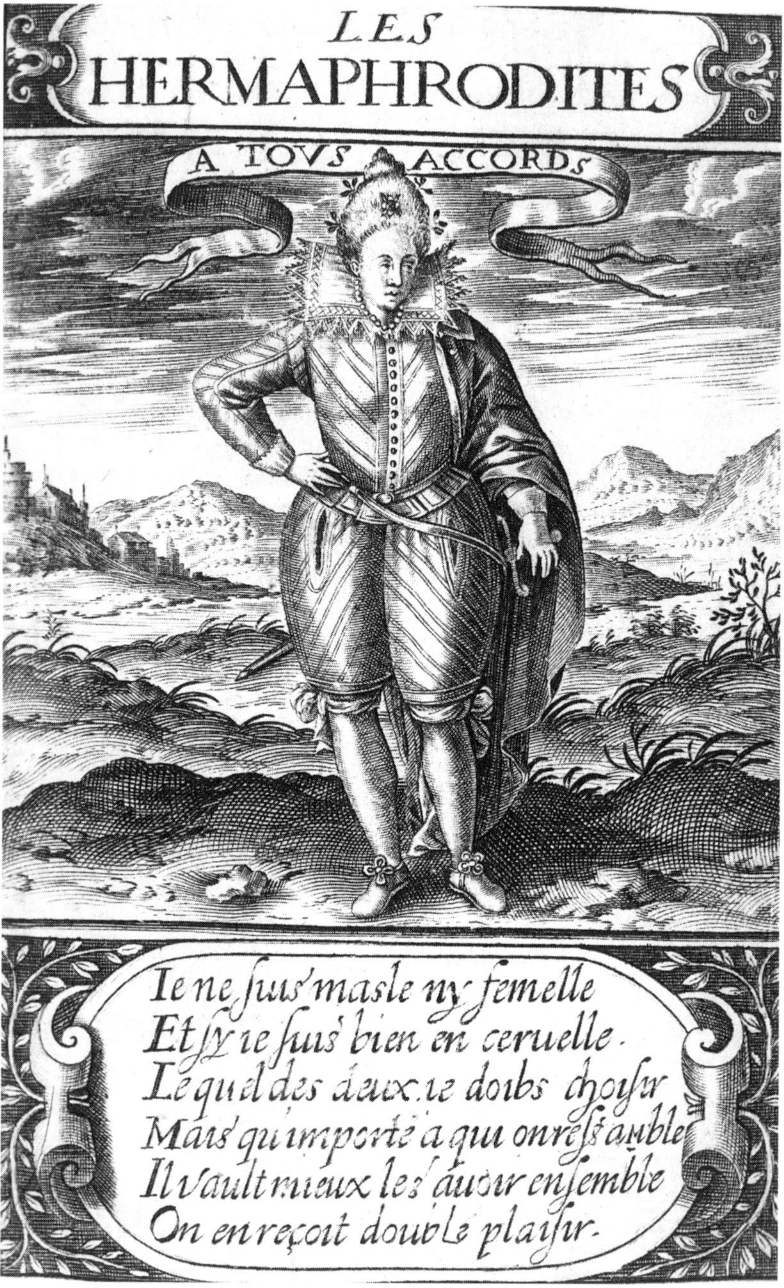

Figure 5.3 Frontispiece from Thomas Artus, *L'Isle des hermaphrodites* (1605). Courtesy of Dartmouth College Library [PQ1601.A8 H4].

In an edition of the *Histoires prodigieuses* from 1597–98, the consequences of gendered hair are even more robustly imagined (Figure 5.2). This figure, which precedes the exact same textual matter, portrays a man who is startlingly resexed and regendered by his hair. While his virile mien (particularly his beard) and his muscular arms denote the vestiges of masculinity, his breasts, full belly, and long flowing locks suggest an entirely female presence. Similar to the earlier edition, the arms are in an outstretched pose of self-display, occasioned here by the man's engagement in the quintessentially feminine activity of spinning. It is as if the man from the earlier edition had been caught in mid-metamorphosis: in this later edition, the true marker of this man's new identity (the distaff) has found its way into his hands; his body has been more radically and roundly reformed (his signature coiffure radiating about him like a fiery halo); and his pose is decidedly more settled and sedentary, retired as he is from the frantic life in transition.

L'Isle des hermaphrodites is likewise preceded by a view of transvestment and gender confusion—a transvestism—that calls all the more attention to itself for being depicted, as in the woodcuts from the *Histoires prodigieuses*, in two modes at once (Figure 5.3). This figure, while stationary, is also displayed frontally, planted in a natural, pastoral setting, shrubs and small trees dotting the immediate landscape with the same mountains and suggestion of dwellings off in the distance as shown in the previous example. This portrait is entirely commensurate with those of Henri III, though one strains to detect the trademark pearls. The portrait is also bifurcated, and in this case the opposing genders read both side to side and top to bottom: the figure's cape drapes amply down the left side, exposing a hand delicately poised on the sword; the elaborately accessorized hair and ruff contrast sharply with the male-coded doublet and breeches. One might remark as well the sword hung diagonally across in the rear (perhaps not inconsequentially) and the prominent slashed pockets on the front that resemble nothing so much as a complement to the phallic business behind. Here again, this vision of confused and excessive gender, literally stitched together, is brought out of the city and into the natural environment that serves so efficiently to mock it. If the woodcuts of "A man with the hair of a woman" does not immediately fortell its connection to its text, the engraving from *L'Isle des hermaphrodites* is quite literally attached: the inscription is placed squarely at the feet of the figure, announcing:

> Ie ne suis masle ny femelle
> Et sy ie suis bien en cervelle
> Lequel des deux ie doibs choisir
> Mais qu'importe a qui on ressamble
> Il vault mieux les avoir ensemble
> On en recoit double plaisir. (Artus 49)
>
> [I am neither male nor female
> And if I am in my right mind
> I must choose one or the other

> But little does it matter which I resemble
> It is better to have them both
> One gets double the pleasure.]

The inscription succinctly underscores the ambiguities of the portrait. While the engraving realizes the overabundance of gender signifiers at least sartorially, the inscription begins by denial: "I am neither nor." Strangely, the figure must make what would appear to be a non-choice: which of these nonentities must he choose to be, if he is in his right mind ("bien en cervelle")? The final three lines quickly contradict the opening, stating that s/he, in fact, has both sexes—not neither—and can receive twice the erotic pleasure. And herein, certainly, lies the fundamental transgression.

Chapter 22 of the *Histoires prodigieuses* is entitled "Histoire prodigieuse d'un monstre du ventre duquel il sortoist un autre homme tout entier, reservé la teste" ["Marvelous story of a monster from whose stomach there emerged another entire man"]. I treat this example as a potentially hermaphroditic figure of a different sort. Typical of this text, the chapter takes its time getting to the main character; the introduction is a discourse on the perils of pleasure:

> Ocellus Lucanus … traictant de la generation, nous enseigne que nous n'allions pas au sacré mariage pour la volupté & plaisir (lequel toutefois n'en peut estre absent) mais que nostre principale intention doit estre de procréer lignée, car les desirs que la divine providence a donnez aux hommes pour la congression, n'ont pas esté ordonnez pour le plaisir seulement, mais pour la perpetuelle conservation & permanence de l'espece. (82)

> [Ocellus Lucanus … writing on reproduction, teaches us that we do not go into marriage for sensual delight or pleasure (which nonetheless cannot be denied) but that our principal intention must be to ensure one's lineage, for the desires that divine providence has accorded men for sexual union are not for pleasure alone, but for the perpetual conservation and permanence of the species.]

Sexual congress was invented by God for the purposes of sustaining human life on the planet, "afin que la terre fust multipliée, les Republiques peuplées, les societez humaines conservées" [so that the Earth be filled, the Republics populated, and human society preserved] (83). What one witnesses in this monster are the fruits of pleasure for pleasure's sake. Typical of discourses on hermaphrodites and monsters is the presumption that they are the product of consorting with either satanic forces or prostitutes: "De telz attouchements illicites naissent quelquefois plusieurs enfantemens monstrueux" [From such illicit encounters are sometimes born various monstrosities] (83). And sure enough, the text reiterates the common wisdom of its time: "Et dit on qu'il avoit esté engendré de quelque femme perdue, qui se prostituoit à tout le monde indifferemment" [And they say that he was born of some fallen woman who prostituted herself wantonly to anyone who would have her] (83). Such are the wages of sexual activity engaged in for purposes other than procreation.

Queer theorist Michael Bronski, among others, has written extensively on the anxiety incurred by unmitigated—read "uncivilized"—enthrallment with Eros. Since homosexual congress, and presumably that of persons undergoing sexual reassignment, offers no issue, it turns back on the pleasure as its only reward—forever and always a dangerous prospect. Bronski's post-Freudian critique of the absence of a repressive, organizing mechanism resulting in civil disorder is not so irrelevant to the moralizing strains of this earlier era.[16] Also instructive in this regard is Mark Jordan's *The Invention of Sodomy in Christian Theology*, which sees the virulence of the condemnation of sodomy as "a displacement of the negative judgment on all sex that was suspended in the case of procreative marriage," and "a failure to think through the problem of the erotic." He concludes:

> To invent Sodomy was to invent a pure essence of the erotic without connection to reproduction. It was to isolate the erotic in its pure state, where it could be described in frightening colors and condemned without concession. "Sodomy" is a name not for a kind of human behavior, but for a failure of theologians to understand how pleasure can survive the preaching of the Gospel.[17]

Boaistuau betrays (and embodies) this failure and this tension quite explicitly: men are seduced by "plaisirs," "attouchement illicites," and women who prostitute themselves with indifference to human dignity—this, in contradistinction with the healthy and perpetual regeneration of the Republic. Of interest is the qualifying language—inserted parenthetically—wherein the author raises the specter of the pleasure to which we are drawn but must never be entirely beholden: "la volupté & plaisir (*lequel toutefois n'en peut estre absent*)" [for sensual delight or pleasure (*which nonetheless cannot be denied*)], and later, the renunciation of the "plaisir *seulement*" [for pleasure *alone*] (my emphases). Herein we witness the inevitable presence and pull of the erotic that is, if not an impulse that dare not speak its name, at best only timidly acknowledged: the pleasure, says Jordan, that can barely—if at all—survive its own telling.[18]

The woodcut at the head of this chapter prepares Boaistuau's disquisition well, again presenting a door (window, tapestry …) through which to interpret his text. I pair it, again, with the version of the same figure from Paré's works to appreciate

---

16 Michael Bronski, *The Pleasure Principle: Sex, Backlash, and the Struggle for Gay Freedom* (New York, 1998), pp. 20, 176.

17 Mark Jordan, *The Invention of Sodomy in Christian Theology* (Chicago, 1997), p. 175.

18 The lack of distinction that I betray here with regard to charges of sodomy and hermaphrodism is, I hope, tolerable, if not a bit dismissive of a range of approaches to the question of diverse sexualities of the period. Aubigné's lumping of these "vices" and a host of others into intolerable behaviors and transgressions in the *Tragiques* is what informs this more generalized taint of debauchery.

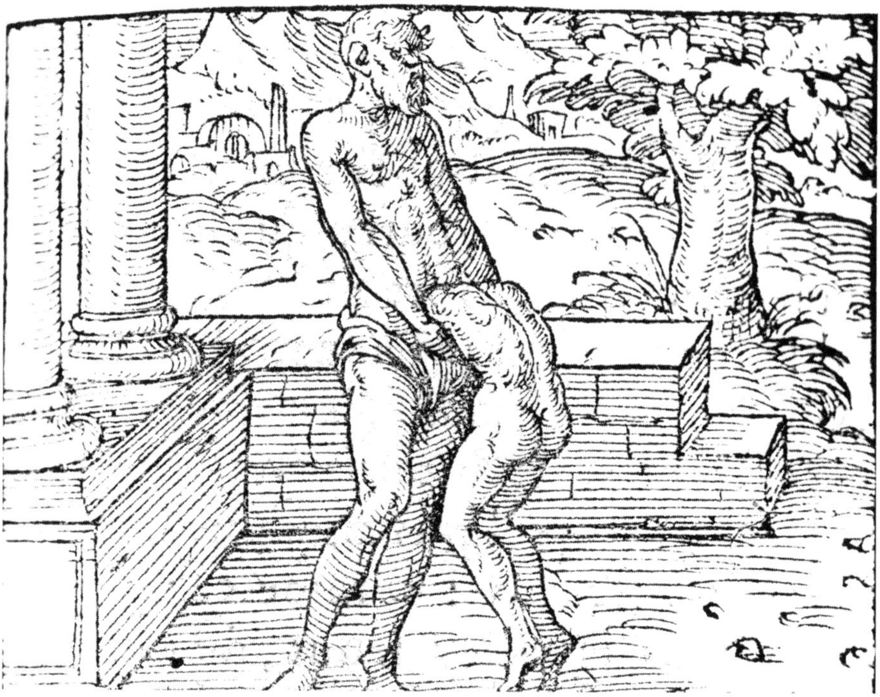

Figure 5.4 Monster from whose belly emerged another man, Pierre Boaistuau, *Histoires prodigieuses* (1597–8). Courtesy of Dartmouth College Library [GR825.B63.1597 v. 1].

the stark difference of this popular figure (like the woman of multiple births) when seen out of cultural and natural contexts (Figures 5.4 and 5.5). While the two versions of the illustration presented here are quite similar, the copy from the *Histoires prodigieuses* (Figure 5.4) relates more closely to the landscapes presented in the previous examples: the monstrous figure stands again in a natural setting with the suggestion of a neoclassical pavilion, the lush natural setting and the civilized hand of the stone architecture contrasting sharply with the hideous grotesque. Nor does the monster have a place in society, referenced by the village in the background from which he may appear to be banished. The figure's nudity suggests an Edenic environment gone awry: his mother's carnal knowledge, pleasure for pleasure's sake, has wrought monstrous consequences.

Boaistuau's text (and subsequent editions) includes several illustrations of hermaphroditic monsters, as do other such works—Ambroise Paré's *Des Monstres et prodiges* [*On Monsters and Marvels*], for example, which borrows a great number of its illustrations from Boaistuau. This illustration is distinct, however, in its composition and what it might suggest for monstrous men of another sort. The man and his conjoined entity—if that is what it is—are not

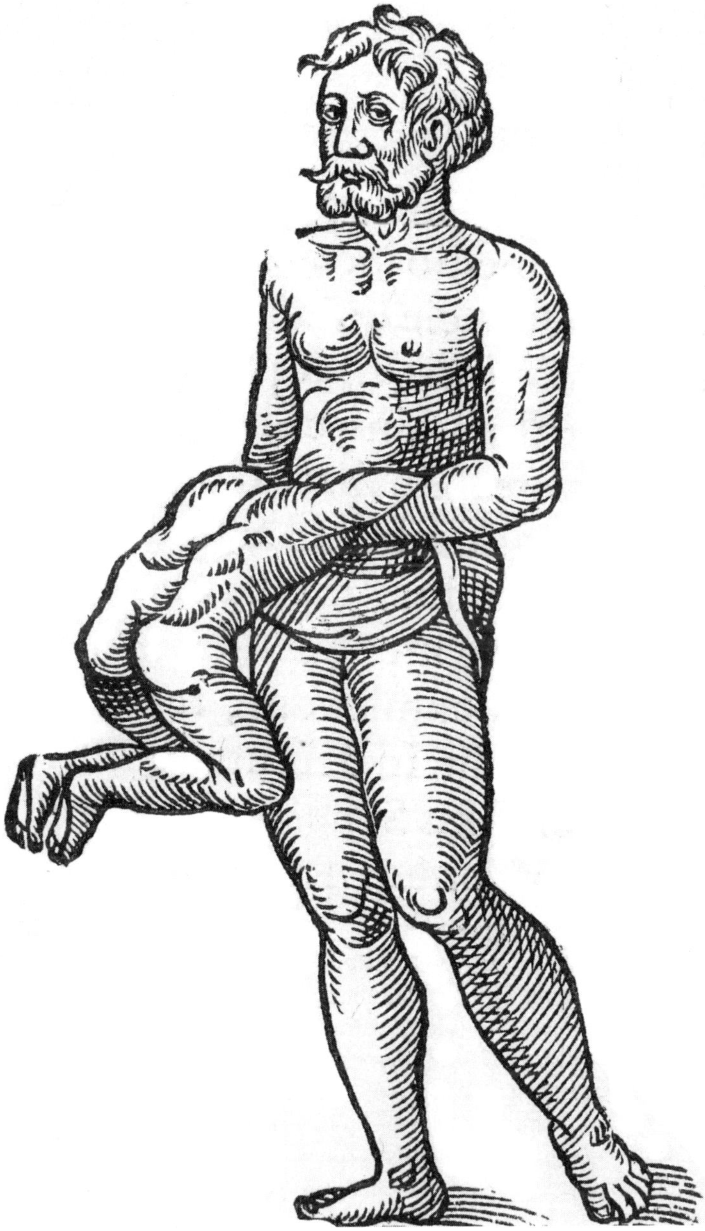

Figure 5.5 Man from whose belly emerged another man, Ambroise Paré, *Les Oeuvres d'Ambroise Paré* (1633). Courtesy of Dartmouth College Library [R128.7 P2 1633].

bifurcated in the manner of the man with a woman's hair, for example, or like Artus's hermaphrodite. The secondary figure extrudes from his midsection, caught, seemingly, in an act of parturition. In the original version, the site of the genitalia is, presumably, draped and hidden (unless, in fact, what appears to be draping is not some representation of ambiguous genitalia). The language of the title seems ambiguous as well: "histoire d'un monstre du ventre duquel il sortait un autre homme" [marvelous story of a monster from whose stomach there emerged another entire man] leaves the agency somewhat unclear, though I favor a reading that suggests that he is actually propelling the other man out of his midsection ("il sortait" can be passive—"there emerged," or active—"he pushed out"). However we wish to interpret this linguistically, visually, the figure bespeaks its own birthing. The beleaguered and condemned man roams the earth as both the monstrosity that he is and also as the embodiment of his generation: the issue of his mother's prostitution, he himself is a monster whose very composition signifies perpetually the diabolical birth in progress.

I would turn, in response, to the beginning of Boaistuau's *Histoire prodigieuses* and consider the image that his readers encounter before entering into his tome of monstrosities (Figure 5.6). Chapter 1, entitled "Prodiges de Sathan," is preceded by a woodcut that furthers this discussion of men and diabolical maternity. Boaistuau's inaugural image (once past the prefatory matter of his work) is of Satan, *en majesté*, in a pose that resembles nothing so much as a woman in childbirth. What is most obvious and central to the viewer—the monstrous head issuing from the site of Satan's genitals—goes surprisingly untreated in the chapter that follows. Boaistuau speaks of two of Satan's most notorious residences, one at the Oracle of Delphi and the other in Calcutta, said to be still in existence at the time of his writing. This is the scene depicted in the woodcut and Boaistuau mentions the throne, the incense, the attendants, the simian hands, and avian feet. The unspoken drama, however, is by far the most remarkable: Satan is possessed of two breasts (more pendulous in other versions) and appears to be pushing out (to borrow the language from the figure we have just left) a monster from between his legs. Boaistuau goes on to illustrate and explicate a host of gynecological monstrosities: this dramatic visualization firmly situates them in the realm of the portentous. Men who consort with prostitutes run with the devil himself and can expect such consequences. This demonic image is the enthronement of the most hyperbolic vision of unstable male bodies imaginable. The prominent, phallic tail descends from the satanic womb; the generous breasts are draped beneath the bearded visage and suggestion of a hairy chest. The throne upon which he sits, the attendants on either side, the columns—all serve to frame the unseemly veneration of this satanic and salacious labor.[19]

---

[19] In the earliest versions of the *Histoires prodigieuses* there is a clear anti-Semitic cast to this engraving as well, where the attendants are unmistakably figured as Jews. For a discussion of this, see Ruth Luborsky (note 15).

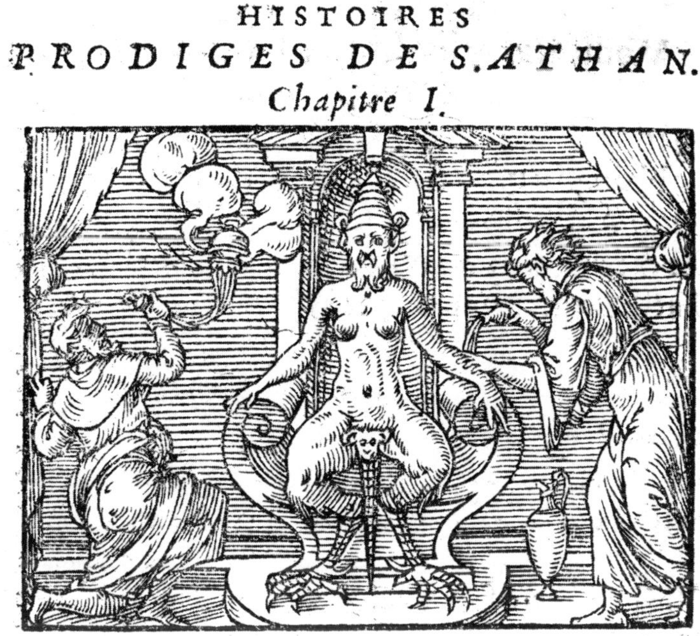

Figure 5.6 Frontispiece, Pierre Boaistuau, *Histoires prodigieuses* (1597–8). Courtesy of Dartmouth College Library [GR825.B63.1597 v. 1].

Two comparative strains of male maternity may have had resonance within the Christian tradition here, and I treat them briefly before discussing some final secular medical and artistic examples from the period. Recent work on the biblical figure Judas Iscariot has brought to light versions of this personnage and an iconography that persistently portray Jesus's betrayer's death as a hideous spectacle of disgorgement and satanic deliverance/delivery. Susan Gubar's monograph compiles compelling illustrations and lore that pair well with Boaistuau's enthroned devil. Of Judas's death, she writes:

> Early stories about the twelfth apostle conflate his moral degeneracy with his physical degeneration … many of the early accounts focused obsessively on his fetid dying. Whether commentators followed Luke, by showing Judas's bowels bursting, or Matthew, by depicting him hanging on a tree, they emphasized stinky deformity, bloating, exploding excrement, bloody intestines, and hemorrhages … Curiously feminized by all these bodily outpourings … [w]hat Judas had nefariously hugged or hoarded to himself during his life … disgorges as he loses control over everything.[20]

[20] Susan Gubar, *Judas: A Biography* (New York, 2009), p. 110.

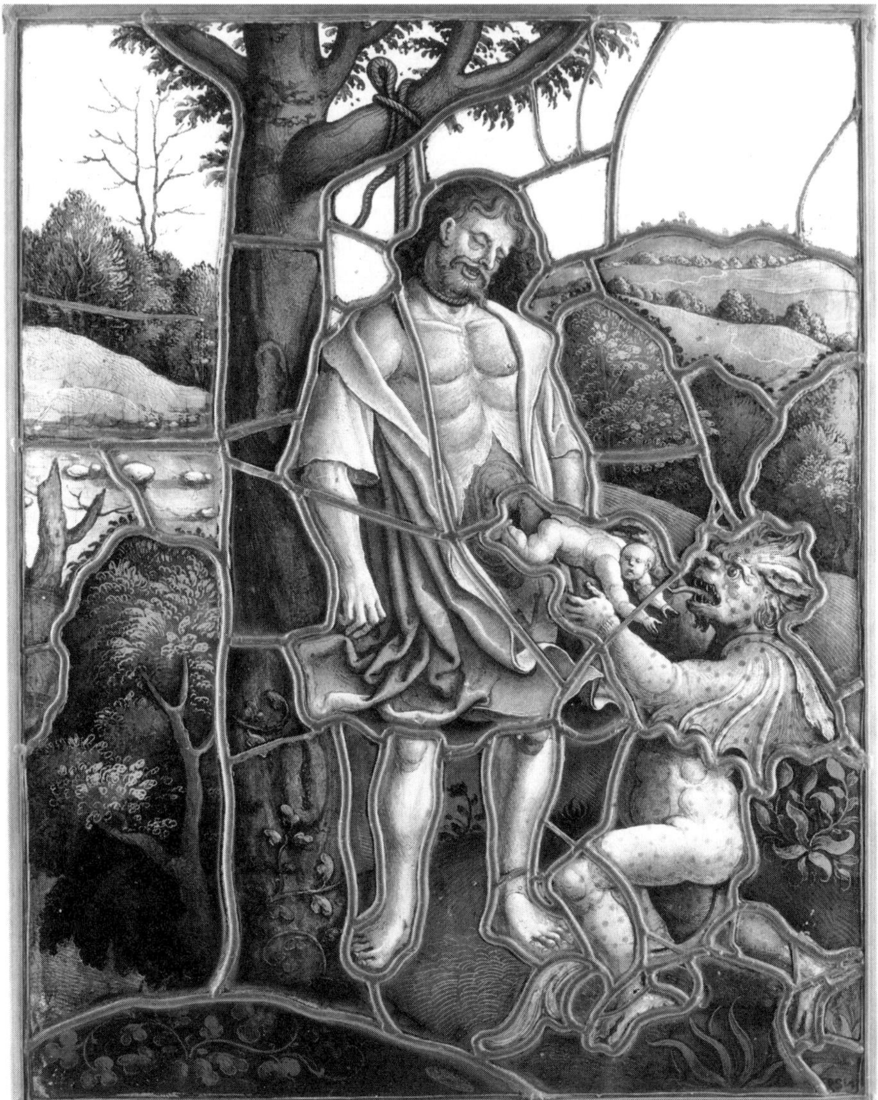

Figure 5.7 *The Hanging of Judas*, Alsatian or southern German (c. 1520). Courtesy of the Art Institute of Chicago.

Several of the early modern depictions that Gubar explores show an infant Judas sprung from his bowels and received by Satan as midwife (Figure 5.7). The Judas figure responds fittingly to the calumny of transvestism and disregard for gender as evinced in Artus and the monstrosities detailed by Boaistuau. Hideous generation seen as disgorgement, disembowelment, and fetid, satanic issue is a dramatic recompense for the sins of Judas that might well be alluded to here with regard to hermaphroditic gender transgressors. By contrast with this iconography of satanic issue there exist more positive maternal male origin stories such as the birth of Eve (springing from the side of Adam) and of the Christian Church itself (Figure 5.8).

Roberto Zapperi speaks of the conflation of these two positive takes on male birthing in his commentary on Christian myth and the pregnant male body:

> The fiction of this "male parturition" acquired a new element of the greatest importance, introduced by the Fathers of the Church. Adam, explained St. Augustine in his Commentary on the Gospel of John, "while he slept, was found

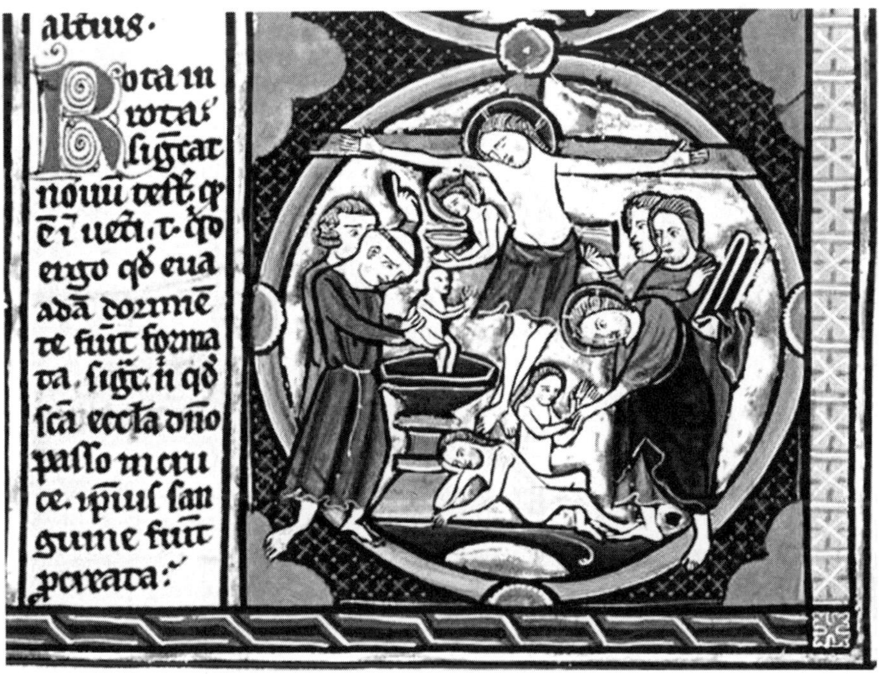

Figure 5.8 Eve emerging from the side of Adam, *Bible moraliste* (thirteenth century). Courtesy of the Bibliothèque Nationale de France [Manuscrits occidentaux, LATIN 11560]

> worthy to receive the wife whom God had formed from his side, because the Church was to be born from Christ as he lay asleep on the Cross, so that from the rib of him who hung upon the Cross pierced by the lance, would flow the Sacraments of the Church."[21]

Both Eve and the Church are thus generated from pregnant men; men in these miraculous situations are given the ability to reproduce when the fate of the world's population and eventual salvation is at stake—no small exception, to be sure. The extent to which these two traditions communicated in the work of Boaistuau is unclear, but such visual and textual narratives existed and had currency in the early modern world. If there were satanic and nefarious versions of the transgendering male figures, there were clearly more felicitous, indeed sacred, employments of the image that perhaps made the darker depictions all the more obvious and deplorable by contrast.[22]

From Monstrous Bodies to Monstrous Texts

Pierre Boaistuau was a compiler and reorganizer of received, sensationalist stories whose subsequent editors and augmenters prized hyperbole and shock over any hint of humanitarian coming to terms with such anatomical curiosities. His contemporary, the doctor Jacques Duval, in his 1612 *Des Hermaphrodits, accouchements des femmes et traitement qui est requis pour les relever en santé* [Of hermaphrodites, women's births and the treatment required for their recovery] is instructive as a rejoinder to the discourse of male mutability and men's prospects in reproduction in the *Histoires prodigieuses*. Duval, as we shall see, while not immune to the titillating impulses of bizarre medical anomalies, presents them with more noble, indeed life-saving motives in mind. Duval tells the story of a young man from the Abbey of Sainte Geneviève who is accused of stealing a silver chalice; the punishment is that he should be stripped naked and whipped in public:

> Oyant ceste sentence prononcee contre luy, il pria qu'on eust compassion de son innocence, & de son sexe, disant qu'il avoit esté garçon & baptisé pour tel, comme de faict il en avoit tousjours porté l'habit, mais depuis quatre à cinq ans il avoit recognu en soy & senty qu'il estoit fille, ce qui seroit manifesté en public, si la sentence portant condemnation du foüet estoit executee.[23]

---

[21] Roberto Zapperi, *The Pregnant Man*, trans. Brian Williams (Chur, 1991), p. 5. See also illustration, p. 6.

[22] The critical work begging inclusion here for a more lengthy treatment is, of course, Caroline Walker Bynum's *Jesus as Mother: Studies in the Spirituality of the High Middle Ages* (Berkeley, 1984).

[23] Jacques Duval, *Des Hermaphrodits, accouchements des femmes et traitement qui est requis pour les relever en santé* (Rouen, 1612), p. 350.

[Hearing this sentence pronounced against him, he begged for mercy based on his naïvety and sex, saying that he had been a boy, and baptized as such, and thus always wore boys' clothing, but during the last four or five years he had recognized in himself and felt that he was a girl—a fact that would be made quite public were the sentence of the public whipping to be carried out.]

The punishment is put off for a time and in the interim the real thief is discovered and hanged; the original suspect is absolved:

Lors ayant esté visité, il fut trouvé avoir une nature féminine bien formee, de laquelle ayant esté raporté qu'il n'avoit abusé, ny mesme d'une petite appendice qu'il avoit en forme de membre viril, au bas de l'os pubis, il luy fut permis prendre l'habit de femme, ce qu'ayant fait, fut joincte par mariage à un Marchand de Vins, dont elle eut enfans. (350)

[When he had been examined, and it was found that he had well-formed feminine parts which, it was reported, he had never touched improperly, and that neither did he abuse himself of a small appendage that had the form of a male member, located at the base of the pubic bone, he was permitted to put on women's clothing, after which he was joined in marriage to a wine merchant with whom she had several children.]

Aside from being a classic case of "l'habit ne fait pas le moine," Duval's narrative says much about the reception and regulation of unstable male bodies. The subject was said to have entered the convent at the age of 12, precisely at the time of the onset of adolescence. In the four or five years since arriving, he recognized his feminine side, as it were. While the instability of the would-be criminal's body is troubling, Duval's rendering suggests that calamity was averted by dint of the subject's lack of sexual indulgence: copious though these genitals may be, none had been "abused." Gender reassignment proceeds with dispatch, so quickly that Duval can switch pronouns even in mid-sentence: *he* has a little male member; *she* has children—the same person, resexed in two short clauses.[24]

Based on other stories from Duval further on, one learns of the high stakes that are at issue with regard to the seclusion of the religious order and its habit for a hermaphroditic adolescent. Ten chapters later, Duval tells "L'Histoire d'une fille-homme à Paris dont le membre viril n'apparoissoit que par intervalles" wherein a "girl" with partially formed male genitals gets to cross over into maleness, with all the rights and privileges pertaining thereto:

---

[24] Butler's evoking of the discourse of the locker room as the modern-day equivalent of the locus of speculation, revelation, and shame comes quickly to mind: "the locker room, that site of prepubescent anxiety about impending gender developments." *Undoing Gender*, p. 63.

> Ce qu'estant suffisamment cognu: le père, après avoir trouvé moyen d'apaiser et pacifier le tout, fit quitter l'habit de fille à ce gunaner, pour prendre l'habit viril, orné duquel il voulut estudier aux lettres humaines, ausquelles il profita si bien en peu de temps, qu'il parvint au cours de Philosophie. (382)
>
> [When all this was discovered, the father, after having found a way to calm everything down, had the girls' clothes removed from his child and put him in men's clothes, and so adorned he wished to study literature; he made out so well in such little time that he went on to courses in Philosophy.]

Here is a clear reminder that sex and gender assignment included not only attitudes and injunctions about sexual pleasure and the primacy of reproductive imperatives, but intellectual livelihood as well. This child's new gender and outfit opened the doors to an academic life of decidedly more glorious and intellectually enriching ends than had he remained in a dress. Maleness was his ticket to a liberal arts education.

Jacques Duval and Pierre Boaistuau (and his accomplices) present two distinct complements to the fiction of Thomas Artus that are linked to their own distinct agendas. Duval's title is perhaps the clearest indication of the way in which he deals with the issue of hermaphrodism and gender instability: *Des Hermaphrodits, accouchemens des femmes et traitement qui est requis pour les relever en santé, et bien élever leurs enfans* [Of hermaphrodites, childbirth, and the required treatment for their care and that of their children] links the question of gender presentation and assignment at birth to health care and proper childrearing. Duval is a doctor whose responsibilities in such questions are practical and official; his observations on hermaphrodites will set the record straight, he tells his readers, concerning what others have said is impossible. Duval's role in this was quite official and indeed decisive, as witnessed in his formative role in the testimony that exonerated Marin de Marcis, a famous hermaphrodite of his time whose sexual ambiguity nearly cost him his life.

Duval proceeds with no little attention to the recognized controversy of his subject matter: procreation is unavoidably, inextricably linked with pleasure and, try as he might, he cannot avoid invoking it in his readers in their act of reading:

> cette exellente ouvriere la puissante nature, desirant beaucoup favoriser, pour tousjours de plus en plus ayder & promouvoir les hommes à la propagation de leur espece … s'est contentee d'exciter une grande delectation, lors que on descend à l'usage d'icelles. Mais aussi elle à par je ne sçay quel instinct, concedé une tant voluptueuse titillation & libidineuse amorce, lors que par la nomination, ou seule signification, l'esprit est attiré à s'y encliner, que quand j'userois de lettres Hierogliphiques empruntees des Egyptiens … encores ne pourrois-je rescinder cette naifve gayeté dont nature à voulu decorer & orner leur commemoration. (iv)

> [this excellent worker, powerful nature, forever hoping to favor and assist in the propagation of the species … afforded a great delectation when one descends to the use of the genitals. But nature has also, by some instinct, allowed such voluptuous titillation and libidinous drive that just by their naming or signification, the spirit is so seduced that were I to use Hieroglyphics borrowed from the Egyptians … to indicate them, I would be powerless to prevent that naïve happiness with which nature has graced and embellished their memory.]

The textual and the sexual are all but one for Duval and while the author wishes to recognize the scandal this might provoke, his obsessive cogitation on the naming of things sexual can be seen as both condemning and flirting with the taint of licentiousness, as witnessed in his rather lengthy fretting over the naming of the virile member.

> Pour le faict des denominations qui luy ont esté données aux autres idiomes, il s'en trouve un tel et si grand nombre, tous significatifs de cette partie, tant entre les Poëtes plus lascifs, vulgaire, maquerelles & putains, que je ne veux tenter de les expliquer, de peur d'offencer le pudique Lecteur. (46)

> [As for the names given to it [the penis] in other idioms, there is to be found so great a number, all signifying this body part, among the most lascivious, base pimping and whoring of poets, that I don't wish even to attempt their explication, for fear of offending the modest Reader.]

Duval's heated prose goes on further in such a way as to suggest the dangers pursuant to even naming the genitals, a risk inherent in the very taxonomy that he must invoke, however trepidatiously, to get at his own medical point.

Duval's mission is, however, profoundly pedagogical, inviting his reader into the experience of the sexual body in a way that has utmost confidence in the power of language:

> J'ay bien voulu contenter les curieux de quelques ratiocinations & arguments pris de la figure, situation & connexion des parties du corps humain, dont tous anatomistes demeurent facilement d'accord, en intention de leur faire toucher quasi du doigt, & veoir comme de l'oeil, qu'en cecy n'y à telle connexité avec l'impossible commes ils estiment. (3)

> [I wished to satisfy those curious about various quibbles and arguments having to do with the shape, the placement, and the connection of the parts of the human body about which the anatomists are largely in agreement, with the intention of allowing the reader to all but touch with their own finger, and see with their very eye, so that by doing so they disabuse themselves of the impossibility of such connections.]

Duval attempts to create an experience whereby his text becomes the direct manifestation of the urgent medical discernments at hand, as it were. And the goal is one of stabilization, as he states in a manner not incommensurate with the first steps of Artus's narrator onto the island of hermaphrodites:

> Car comme celuy qui marche, doit de necessité appuyer fermement un pied sur quelque chose solide, pour ayant haussé l'autre en l'air, en l'advançant ou retirant arriere, faire tel progrez qu'il advisera bon estre. (3)
>
> [For like he who walks, one must necessarily plant one's foot firmly upon something solid, for having lifted the other up to move forward or backward, in order to make progress.]

To paraphrase Bordo, Duval seems acutely aware of the commitments that the hermaphroditic body is inscribing and enforcing and which, not inconsequentially, obtain to his very own text. Would that his writing that can "make us all but touch with our own finger," not lead him and us to perdition: a monstrous text born from a monstrous subject.

Boaistuau's text makes this ever more explicit. In his lengthy, turgid dedicatory preface to Jean de Rieux, to whom he hands over his stories, he describes his subject as follows:

> Accidens estranges, & prodigieux evenemens, desquels toutes les provinces du monde ont esté espouventees depuis la nativité de Jesus Christ jusques à nostre siecle. Or maintenant Monseigneur que j'ay combatu avec le labeur, & qu'à mon advis je suis sorty victorieux, il ne me reste autre chose pour le parfaict accomplissement de mes desseings, que de vous offrir, consacrer & dedier ce fruict abortif de mes muses, & juste tribut de mes peines. (Boaistuau 3)
>
> [Strange accidents, prodigious events about which all corners of the world have been horrified since the birth of Jesus Christ to the current century. Now, my Lord, that I have battled in labor, and (in my opinion) emerged victorious, the perfect realization of my plans requires only that I offer, consecrate, and dedicate to you this abortive (premature?) fruit of my muses, a worthy tribute of my pains.]

Boaistuau's mission is not a medical one; as a man who made his name as a compiler, editor, and writer (the inventor, some say, of the popular *genre* of *histoires prodigieuses*), he aimed to create a sensational text, a work that is, he freely admits, a compendium of shocking and hideous events, all framed—as was made evident from the first chapter, "Les prodiges de Sathan"—as an act of birthing.[25]

[25] See in this regard Jean Céard's thorough-going treatment of Boaistuau and his contemporaries, especially *La Nature et les prodiges* (Geneva, 1977), Chapter X, "Les Débuts d'un genre: l'histoire prodigieuse (1560)."

His discourse here is replete with birth and labor, from the miraculous virgin birth of Jesus through to the present day. But will he and his text escape calumny? He has wrestled in labor, he has emerged victorious—a birthing metaphor as well—and he offers his text as the aborted fruits of this labor: Boaistuau presents a sort of Chinese box of labors issuing from labors, texts birthing texts. Men birthing monstrosities is titillatingly close to the hideous examples he is about to expose.

Curiously, this act of monstrous redaction was a travesty of which Pierre Boaistuau had been recently accused. I refer here to the immense consternation over his highly controversial edition of Marguerite de Navarre's *Heptameron*. If Boaistuau's name lives on today it is, for many, primarily for his role in the initial publication of Marguerite's novellas in 1558, two years prior to the *Histoires prodigieuses*. Boaistuau's truncating, reordering, and "cleaning up" of Marguerite's work, which he entitles *Histoires des amans fortunez*, with but veiled attribution to the author herself, persists, let us say, as an undeniably monstrous act of appropriation and misrepresentation, even given the more forgiving standards of imitation and inventive license of the time. As Nancy Virtue has observed, "one cannot help but find it, if not 'strange,' at least ironic that a work in which images of sexual violation recur with haunting frequency should itself undergo such a strident textual violation."[26] Boaistuau's "botched" edition was quickly suppressed by Jeanne d'Albret (Marguerite's daughter) and recommissioned to Claude Gruget; as a result of this high-profile scandal, Boaistuau lost his position as secretary to François de Clèves and lives on in quiet infamy to this day for his role in bringing Marguerite's now famous and beloved work to light in such monstrous fashion (Virtue 35–7). Thus, the literal and literary notions of unstable men's "issue" are conflated: the hermaphroditic, the monstrous hybrid haunts and sullies the life and livelihood of those who would even speak its name, a textual and sexual conundrum of no little consequence and an obvious source of anxiety.

Mitigating Monstrosity

But what of the possibility that hermaphrodism might not finally and always denote the corruption of the human species, that the bodies that defy the norm of a binary sex/gender universe might actually have had a currency of their own and mitigated against this oppression in small, albeit important ways? I conclude this discussion of the putatively monstrous male body with two mediating painterly examples in circulation during this period, along with some observations from the present-day discourse on intersexuality and transgenderism. First, Jusepe de Ribera's *Magdalena Ventura with Her Husband and Son*, painted from life in 1631 (Figure 5.9). Ribera was a well-known Spanish painter living in Naples (then controlled

[26] Nancy E. Virtue, "Translation as Violation: A Reading of Pierre Boaistuau's *Histoires tragiques*," *Renaissance and Reformation/Renaissance et Réforme*, 22/3 (1998): p. 36.

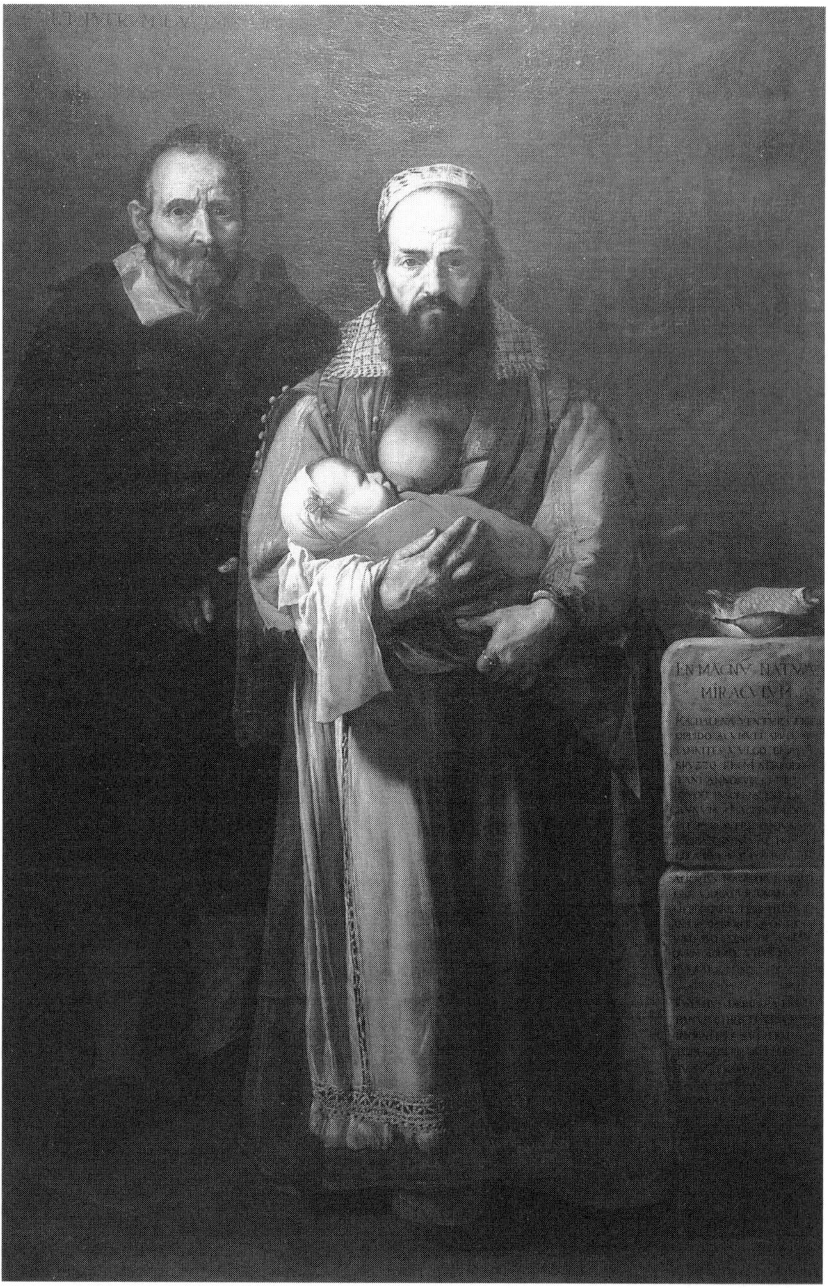

Figure 5.9 *Magdalena Ventura with Her Husband and Son*, Jusepe de Ribera (1651). Courtesy of Fundación Casa Ducal de Medinaceli.

by Spain) who benefited greatly from the patronage of Fernando Afán de Ribera y Enriquez, Duke of Alcalá, who commissioned this painting.[27] This arresting family portrait shares with the hermaphrodite engraving from Artus's text a bold frontal composition, an inscription (here engraved on a plinth to the right), and meticulous attention to sartorial detail. If the hermaphrodite is but a lone figure in Artus, here the gender narrative is accomplished in three persons. The markers of Magdalena's femininity are clearly her dress, the child in her arms (described as her very own) and, of course, the full, round breast protruding somewhat improbably—at best, awkwardly—from the center of her chest. Her son's lips meeting her nipple are the very central, focal point of the portrait. The rest of her person and her husband stand in marked contrast: her receding hairline, her weathered masculine visage, her long beard falling onto the hirsute upper chest, the suckling child cradled in large (oversized?) hands which frame and support him. The husband, utterly and unambiguously masculine-coded, stands in his wife's shadow, staring, like his wife, though somewhat more wearily, directly at the viewer. The inscription boldly announces: EN MAGNUM NATURAE MIRACULUM, "Great Wonder of Nature." The rest pertains mainly to the artist and his various attributes, but does offer Magdalena's age—52—and the age at which she began her curious, bodily transformation—37: "She began to become hairy and grew a beard so long and thick that is seems more like that of any bearded gentleman than of a woman who had borne three sons by her husband, Felici de Amici, whom you see here." The portrait is thus thoroughly imbued with masculinity: Magdalena has been transformed, her husband stands by her, and the child in her arms is but one of three sons. It would appear a masculinist conspiracy for reproductive domination.

We see hints of the woodcuts from the *Histoires prodigieuses*: the frontality of the "man with women's hair," its self-conscious self-exposure prompted like Ribera with declarative hands. Also conversant with this portrait might be the "Monster from whose belly emerged another (entire man)": both masculine figures cradling the issue of their "monstrous" bodies. If the portrait from the *Histoires prodigieuses* presents the subject's alienation by the unseemly contrast between the classically rendered pavilion in the bucolic natural setting that serve to mock him (Figure 5.4)—and we remember as well the similar setting of the latter version of "Man with the hair of a woman" (Figure 5.2)—Magdalena stands firmly in her dress, in her home with her child, defying the incongruity of her apparent gender.[28] And this would be perhaps the less monstrous, more generous view of unstable male-coded bodies that one might impart. Ribera, as observed, presents the scene with neither horror nor judgment: Magdalena is presented not as a monster, but a miracle of nature.

Will Fisher's thorough and illuminating work on the beard's currency in this period includes lengthy commentary on Ribera's portrait that suggests that the term

[27] See *Jusepe de Ribera: lo Spagnoletto 1591–1652* (Fort Worth, 1982), pp. 129–31.

[28] The other equally jarring presentation is the same figure in Paré's text, where the figure (as with the very pregnant woman) floats on the page without any suggestion of a cultural or natural context that might (or could) contain it.

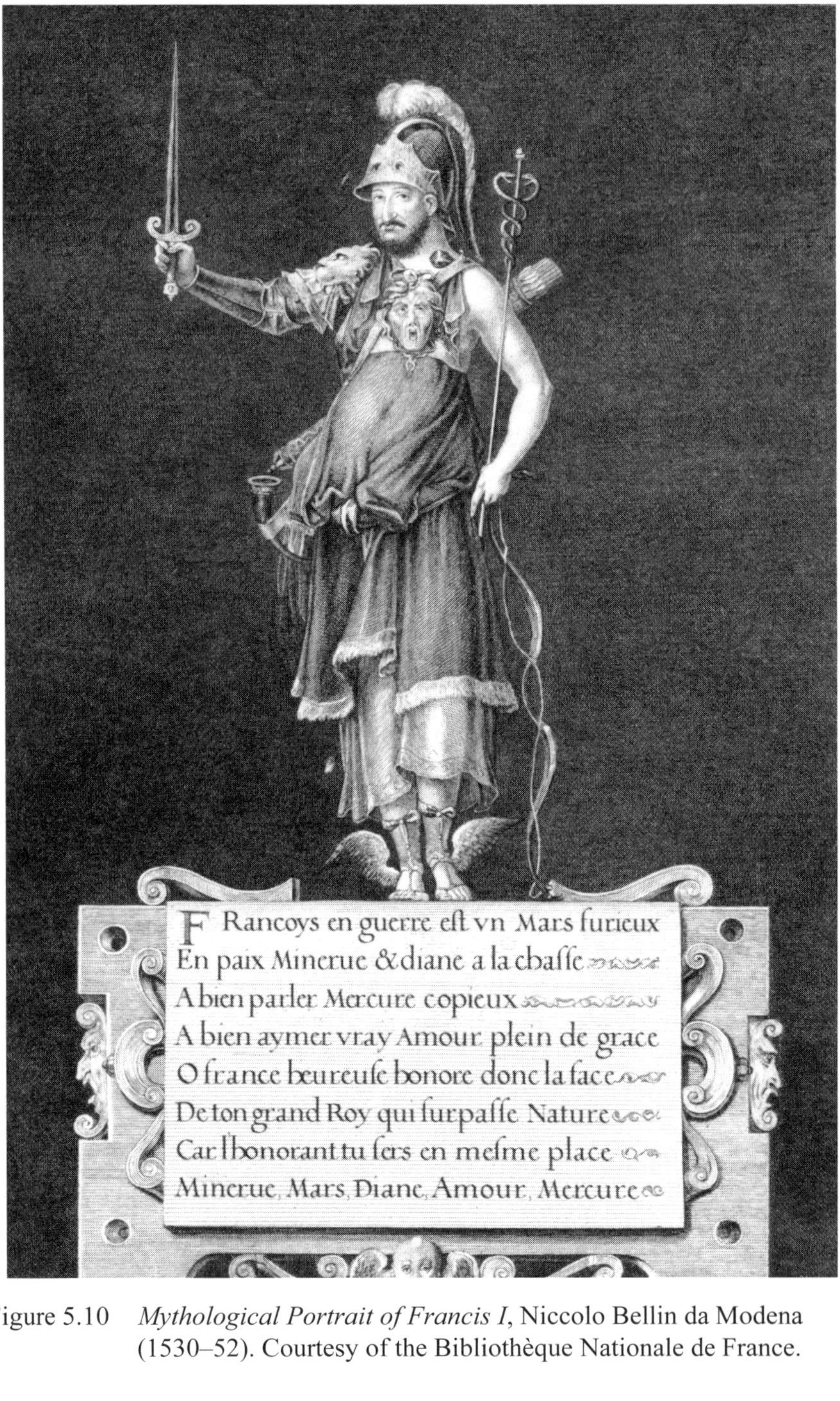
FRancoys en guerre eſt vn Mars furieux
En paix Minerue & diane a la chaſſe
A bien parler Mercure copieux
A bien aymer vray Amour plein de grace
O france heureuſe honore donc la face
De ton grand Roy qui ſurpaſſe Nature
Car lhonorant tu ſers en meſme place
Minerue, Mars, Diane, Amour, Mercure

Figure 5.10 *Mythological Portrait of Francis I*, Niccolo Bellin da Modena (1530–52). Courtesy of the Bibliothèque Nationale de France.

"bearded lady," while controversial, need not be read as oxymoronically as expected. Indeed, Magdalena's hirsuteness is arresting and Fisher reads the array of "feminine" accessories in the portrait as perhaps heavily compensatory, "a testament to the symbolic power of the beard—an indication of the massive cultural work which must be done in order to offset it."[29] Fisher complicates this highly determined "constitutive element of gendered identity," however, by positing that hairiness was not the exclusive domain of men. He asks why Ribera would have said that Magdalena's beard is "*more* like that of any bearded gentleman *than of a woman*," suggesting that it is not the absence or presence of facial hair but the relative amount that registers one's gender (172). Fisher also goes on to investigate the ways in which the beard was not necessarily most valued as a marker of gender but of age, separating boys from men. In the end, it is Magdalena's (and Ribera's) unapologetic witness to her unconventional embodiment of gender that is most arresting. She (and her husband, it must be said) stand in defiance of the potential calumny that her physiognomy might well incur, a reproductive body that demands a more capacious view of its gender.[30]

I would consider the Ribera portrait alongside the famous "androgynous" or "bisexual" (see characterizations to come) portrait of Francis I, attributed variously to Niccolò Bellin da Modena or Niccolò dell'Abbate, painted between 1530 and 1552 (Figure 5.10).[31] The portrait contrasts sharply with more official, unabashedly virile representations—the Clouet from the 1520s and the 1539 Titian, for example.

---

[29] Will Fisher, "The Renaissance Beard: Masculinity in Early Modern England," *Renaissance Quarterly*, 54/1 (2001): p. 171.

[30] While documented reactions to the painting of the period elude us, contemporary descriptions from interested parties speak forcefully to its perceived transgression. From the entry on Ribera in the Catholic online encyclopedia, *New Advent* (http://www.newadvent.org/cathen/13031b.htm):

> No one demonstrates so well the profound change which took place in men's minds after the Reformation and the Council of Trent. Thenceforth concern for character and accent forestalled every other consideration. Leanness, weariness, and abasement became the pictorial signs of the spiritual life … Search for character became that of ugliness and monstrosity. Nothing is so personal to Ribera as this love of deformity. Paintings like … the "Bearded Woman" inaugurate curiosities which had happily been foreign to the spirit of the Renaissance. They show a gloomy pleasure in humiliating human nature. Art, which formerly used to glorify life, now violently emphasized its vices and defects. The artist seized upon the most ghastly aspects even of antiquity … This artistic terrorism won for Ribera his sinister reputation, and it must be admitted that it had depraved and perverted qualities.

Here we see the realization of Boaistuau's nightmare, as the hideous immorality of the subject attaches itself to its author's reputation: depraved and perverted progeny can only issue from depraved and perverted artists.

[31] For purposes of reproduction, I have chosen the contemporaneous engraving of the portrait by P. Chenu (also at the Bibliothèque Nationale de France).

In keeping with the representations of unstable and unclassifiable bodies assembled thus far, the portrait leads in multiple directions, side to side and top to bottom. The curve of the milky, descending, naked left arm responding to the upraised, armored, sword-bearing right; the crested helmet over the bearded visage sculpted onto a torso whose full, round belly anchors the portrait: if this is not a pregnant body, it certainly appeals to Renaissance notions of female corpulent grace and fecundity. The inscription explicates the various and sundry mythological accoutrements that Francis enjoys, from the winged feet to the armor and quiver; he is become a composite god: "en mesme place Minerve, Mars, Diane, Amour, Mercure" [at once Minerva, Mars, Diana, and Mercury] as the inscription tells us. The portrait is stunning for this dizzying array of signifiers and enjoys a reception that is, perhaps fittingly, ambiguous. Raymond Waddington begins by interpreting the portrait in contrast to its reworking several decades later into a portrait of Francis's son, Henri II: the debt that the medallion of Henri's portrait owes to the androgynous original is clear and convincing; the evolution is a curious case of restabilization of the male body. Says Waddington,

> Far from appearing with a woman's body and dress, this king is a battle-ready commander with a man's body in a neutral costume, already partially stripped to fight. This icon of military leadership presents a thoroughly masculine figure with two almost incidental and hardly recognizable attributes of feminine divinities, breastplate and hunting horn. The artist has performed a successful sex-change operation on Bellin da Modena's monstrously bisexual Francis I.[32]

Like the erstwhile Heliogabalus, who attempts a torturous sex transformation that leaves him neither nor, Waddington's Francis I is a post-op monstrosity; Henri II is the post-op poster boy, all of the signs of his unwelcome ambiguity cleanly excised. Waddington's analysis of the portrait proceeds to temper this "monstrosity" by proposing that Francis I may well have tolerated this (what he sees as comical) portrait as a sign of his grace and noble magnanimity: Francis I playing to the tradition of the laughing or witty ruler, a role he inhabited more fully, Waddington posits, thanks to his association with Castiglione. Barbara Meyer's reading of the portrait eschews the comical and interprets the king as *appealingly* androgynous; she proposes that the work was commissioned by Marguerite to reflect her love for her brother: the feminine and masculine elements in this portrait are interpreted by Meyer as the Neoplatonic conflation

---

32 Raymond B. Waddington, "The Bisexual Portrait of Francis I: Fontainebleau, Castiglione, and the Tone of Courtly Mythology," in Jean Brink, Maryanne C. Horowitz, and Allison P. Coudert (eds), *Playing with Gender: A Renaissance Pursuit* (Chicago, 1991), p. 105.

of the king and his adoring sister.[33] The portrait circulates as an "appropriate expression of Marguerite's love for her brother," a symbol of their reunification after her banishment following the "affaire des placards," and, nonetheless, a still somewhat vexed negotiation between the carnality and spirituality evident in Marguerite's heady *homages* to Francis in the *Miroir* and *Navire* poetic cycles. Kathleen P. Long, in weighing the various interpretations of this unique portrait, asks a question that is both crucial and generous. In that the portrait clearly responds to contemporaneous poetic concerns, she asks:

> And why shouldn't poetry based on the hermaphrodite be strangely dualistic in nature, offering conflicting possibilities in the same representation, dualities that cannot be reconciled or subsumed into the greater whole, just as the hermaphrodite cannot be made to conform to merely one sex, or even to the general schema of sexual difference? (Long 200)

Indeed. The question and/or accusation of hermaphrodism is best turned back on its own defining feature, ambiguity, though not as a reenactment of that accusation, but as an exploration and opening of non-binary, non-normative ways of being in the world. As Kessler admonishes us, as arbiters and constructors of both sex and gender and the system that sustains them, we seem forever wont to "correct" for ambiguity and codify as monstrous the "incorrect" or non-normative. These final portraits may serve as instructive counter-examples.

The story that Thomas Artus's island explorer confronts on the tapestry that both shrouds and explicates the mysteries of hermaphrodism through the example of Heliogabalus is horrific. This chapter has suggested that while some contemporaneous depictions of unstable or ambiguously gendered bodies evince this same horror, others do not. Some subjects willfully accepted and displayed their indeterminacy. While Ribera may well have sought Magdalena Ventura out for her "miraculous" qualities, it does seem significant that his subject did little to dissemble the signs of her masculine encroachment: she could have shaved, disguised her receding hairline, softened her features in a such a way as to suggest more conventional womanhood. Likewise, the fictional "man with the hair of a woman," who remains unexplicated but for this brief, tantalizing descriptor, could have cut his hair: there is nothing in the literature of the period to indicate notions of feminine or masculine hair other than length. The portrait of Francis I was not, to anyone's knowledge, roundly condemned or censored.[34] The evidence gleaned for this chapter suggests that unstable bodies of this period, bodies in transition or in states that defied convention, may have had a value beyond horror or monstrosity.

---

[33] Barbara Hochstetler Meyer, "Marguerite de Navarre and the Androgynous Portrait of François Ier," *Renaissance Quarterly*, 48/2 (1995): p. 288.

[34] As evidence of the portrait's appeal, it is interesting to see it featured (without commentary) as the only likeness of Francis I in the official, illustrated timeline at the Bibliothèque Nationale de France.

They may well open up the discourse of the past to a generosity with regard to human potential that is at once revelatory and salutary.

To extend this discussion of gender ambiguity as calamitous, ruinous or, as in the case of these last examples, more accepting even in their curiosity and exceptionality, I would point to the emphasis in contemporary discussions of early modern gender and the persistent evocation of anxiety. Reeser's work, *Moderating Masculinity*, relies on the tensions of normative and aberrant as an anxious discourse in male self-conception and mastery; the anthology *High Anxiety: Masculinity in Crisis in Early Modern France* (2002) announces this tension quite baldly and offers a range of responses that are frequently gender-inflected; and finally Mark Breitenberg's *Anxious Masculinity in Early Modern England* (1996) explores this emotion at length. He posits:

> Masculinity is inherently anxious: according to this argument, anxiety is not a secondary effect of masculinity, nor simply an unpleasant aberration from what we might hypothetically understand as normative. Instead, I argue that masculine anxiety is a necessary and inevitable condition that operates on at least two significant levels: it reveals the fissures and contradictions of patriarchal systems and, at the same time, it paradoxically enables and drives patriarchy's reproduction and continuation of itself.[35]

Breitenberg's convincing thesis is that patriarchy and anxiety go hand in hand; anxiety is constitutive of masculinity, embedded, necessary and, as he makes clear throughout his work, productive. He sees the early modern period as particularly agitated and restive (17), with disruption of gender norms and particularly of family as a constant source of anxiety. I have shown as well the ways in which this anxiety is witnessed and performed in the highly self-conscious narratives in which the tales of monstrosity are embedded: both Duval and Boaistuau fret in their prefatory rhetoric about the potential monstrosity of their body of writing—a sort of guilt by association that we saw witnessed in Guillemeau's anonymous translator in Chapter 3. There but for the grace of God (and a gentle reader) go they, their curious texts no less horrifying than the satanic birth; or the inert, half-formed twin issuing from the beleaguered man's midsection; or the inscrutable composites of male and female stuck out in nature (to announce all the more efficiently their status *out* of nature). Yet I hope to have suggested without overreaching, the "fissures and contradictions," to quote Breitenberg, through which a moderating, less anxious response may have existed: the young convent boy-become-girl whose transition through gender was survivable; Duval, the doctor, who appeared to have his human interests at heart; a popular portrait of the most conventionally virile and masculine king (Francis I) as a gendered composite with multiple readings and

---

[35] Kathleen P. Long (ed.), *High Anxiety: Masculinity in Crisis in Early Modern France* (Kirksville, 2002); Mark Breitenberg, *Anxious Masculinity in Early Modern England* (Cambridge, 1996), p. 2.

assessments; and the stunning portrait of Magdalena Ventura, whose exceptional appearance did not condemn her prospects. Indeed the pose that is chosen for the family portrait (the child held to an exaggeratedly full, rotund, and centrally positioned breast) exemplifies her ability to nourish a vision of family that, though seemingly unconventional, references nothing so much as the iconography of the Virgin Mother herself. Such is a view to patriarchy's "reproduction of itself" (again, Breitenberg) that suggests an early modern capaciousness with regard to sex and gender assignment that may be instructive.

In conclusion, our exploration is well complemented by contemporary inquiry by and about intersexual and transgendering persons. It is a discourse that revalues the purportedly unstable body that heteronormative cultures have perennially worked so hard to codify into a binary sexual universe. The anxieties created by sexual ambiguity are made manifest in the most immediate of ways; the tapestry is pulled back by the subjects themselves and we are shown the monstrosity not only of the hermaphroditic body, but also of the forces that would not abide by their perceived inscrutability. Cheryl Chase, an intersexual scholar and activist whose body was resexed for her as a child, reminds us that:

> The insistence on two clearly distinguished sexes has calamitous personal consequences for the many individuals who arrive in the world with sexual anatomy that fails to be easily distinguished as male or female … Pediatric genital surgeries literalize what might otherwise be considered a theoretical operation: the attempted production of normatively sexed bodies and gendered subjects through constitutive acts of violence.[36]

The operative and recurrent theme employed in the discourse on intersexuality is violence. Artus, Boaistuau, and Duval clearly betray the anxiety of this violation, explicating, fearing, and sometimes enacting it, as the legacy of Boaistuau's work illustrates. Transgender activist Sandy Stone both announces and complicates what is at stake in Chase's account, a debate she describes as "the battlefield of the transsexual body: a hotly contested site of cultural inscription, a meaning machine for the production of ideal type."[37] The transsexual body becomes a text, "a story which culture tells itself … a tactile politics of reproduction constituted through textual violence. The clinic is a technology of inscription" (350). Stone warns against the erasure of one's past that occurs in the transition of many transgendering and transsexualizing individuals; "passing" becomes the eradication of memory and the disappearance into "plausible histories":

---

[36] Cheryl Chase, "Hermaphrodites with Attitude: Mapping the Emergence of Intersex Political Activism," *Journal of Lesbian and Gay Studies*, 4/2 (1998): p. 189.

[37] Sandy Stone, "The Empire Strikes Back: A Posttranssexual Manifesto," in Conboy, Medina, and Stanbury, *Writing on the Body*, p. 350.

> The most critical thing a transsexual can do, the thing that constitutes success, is to "pass." Passing means to live successfully in the gender of choice, to be accepted as a "natural" member of that gender. Passing means the denial of mixture … [T]his process forecloses the possibility of a life grounded in the intertextual possibilities of the transsexual body. (352)

What of the panoply of intersexual "monstrosities" displayed in these texts, both literary and pictorial? The satanic labor that so graphically introduces Boaistuau's book of marvels calls us dramatically into not only the fear of the intersexual being itself, but also of our way of speaking it, of birthing it. For the "marvels of Satan," are both a collection of curiosities and a discourse. What these unstable bodies are and how we speak of them are of a piece. Like the monster birthing its own monstrous progeny, our discourse may well reveal and judge both author and subject. Such was the fear of Boaistuau and Duval. Allowing our gaze and our discourse to live fully in the transitional space is perhaps the way out of monstrosity. Stone advises us that it is the fullness of these subjects past and present, inscribed in all of their complexity, that will teach us the most about our own capacity to imagine a non-binary sexual universe.

Judith Butler's treatment of the tragic case of "David," who lived a life far more regulated and circumscribed than, say, our case of the accused boy/girl in the convent, or, from all evidence, Magdalena Ventura and her husband, ends by privileging the voice of the subject himself, whose narrative about his life pleads for a lovability and acceptability that is "not reducible to the compatibility of his anatomy and the norm." "Something exceeds the norm, and he recognized its unrecognizability" (Butler 72). This gender outlier furthermore, and finally, cautions against the absolutism of distinction itself, a lament against a socio-medical establishment that would prize him and define him so solely on the recognizability of what is found between his legs (72). As is clear from the body narratives of this chapter (and of much of this book), the self-controlled story of such people is rare; we would be wise to read the stories of monstrosity, ambiguity, and sexual confusion with an eye on the regulators and their conventions—literary, political, and/or medical—and their power to determine comprehensibility and acceptability. There is evidence to suggest that the early modern era betrayed both the rigidity and the flexibility with regard to such ambiguity as our present-day examples; in retelling these stories with attention to such "regulation," perhaps the specter of instability that so roils in our present discourse can become less monstrous, less binary, and more generous to both the past and future.

Chapter 6
Strange Fellows in Bed: Exotic Men's Postpartum Blues

> But what is really initiated here is a colonization of the body by the discourse of power. This is writing that conquers. It will use the New World as if it were a blank, "savage" page on which Western desire will be written. It will transform the space of the other into a field of expansion for a system of production.[1]
>
> Michel de Certeau, *The Writing of History*

In this final chapter, we return to Chapter 2 to revisit the births depicted in Rabelais's gargantuan tales and the text that inspired them. As we recall, the *Grandes cronicques* (Rabelais's text of origin) presents the labor of birth as shared between the parents Gargamelle and Grandgousier; in fact, while there is no actual description of Gargamelle's labor—she falls behind on their hunting adventure and Grandgousier turns back to find that she has already given birth without him—it is the *father* whose Herculean labor stands in for hers. His reenactment of the capture of the Hind of Ceryneia, a labor of mythological proportions, supplants that of Gargamelle, whose travails transpire unwitnessed and untold. In this version, Gargantua's nativity is as quiet and unspectacular as the Rabelaisian version is raucous and outrageous. Our reading of the postpartum settings in Rabelais, particularly in *Pantagruel*, further suggested a masculinized birth chronicle wherein Gargantua (here the father) takes to childbed in grief over his wife's passing and attends to his son's first moments in the world: "Go to her burial," he implores the attendants, "I'll rock my baby son right here, for I feel quite parched, and might be in danger of falling ill" [allez à l'enterrement d'elle, et ce pendent je berceray icy mon filz, car je me sens bien fort alteré, et serois en danger de tomber malade].[2]

Brooding Men

This scene of unusual postpartum paternity is known as "couvade," and recurs in a variety of narrative accounts over time in surprisingly similar ways; the etymology of the term is the French "couver," or to brood. The couvade, while not a deeply

---

[1] Michel de Certeau, *The Writing of History* (New York, 1988), p. xv.

[2] François Rabelais, *Oeuvres complètes*, ed. Mireille Huchon (Paris, 1994), pp. 226. Translation: Donald M. Frame, *The Complete Works of François Rabelais* (Berkeley, 1991), p. 144. All other translations are my own unless otherwise noted.

researched phenomenon, has been reported since antiquity and recurs in accounts of various societies, most often in ethnographic or anthropological literature as a custom that serves to exoticize cultures perceived of as distinctly other or barbarous. The most comprehensive contemporary study, Warren Dawson's *The Custom of the Couvade* (1929), is problematic in ways that have everything to do with my thesis regarding the couvade practice and the depiction of New World culture. Dawson traces the couvade across multiple centuries and rather breezily across cultures. Commenting upon the birthing practices among many couvade societies, he observes: "In the first place, the pains of childbirth amongst primitive peoples are not necessarily serious; the birth of a child to such a mother is not normally the prostrating and anxious crisis that befalls her civilized sisters."[3] Such racist and ethnocentric observation is altogether consistent with the accounts I consider for comparison in this chapter. The assumptions regarding "developing" or "Third World" women's comparatively easy labor and birthing are taken up later as complementary discourse when speaking of the bizarre behaviors of their postpartum menfolk. In worlds upside down, it appears, mothers' labors in childbed are as easy as the fathers' are arduous and painful.

Couvade is also reported and investigated in the modern era as a psychological phenomenon, though no official treatment is reported as yet in official diagnostic manuals. Of the limited literature on the couvade in the field of psychology, Hilary Klein delineates several strains of thought that mark this phenomenon in distinct ways. Klein reviews the earlier work of Dawson and others, followed by more contemporary theories under the following rubrics: identification with the expectant mother, ambivalence about fatherhood, fetus as rival, roots of fatherliness, sexuality and gender identity issues, parturition envy, and defense against aggressive impulses.[4] While I do not take up the task of repermutating these more modern—and, I would argue, highly Eurocentric—psychodynamic approaches in the context of the early modern reporting of couvade, I hold some of them in mind as I analyze what is at play in the protocolonialist gestures of these early explorers and reporters. In my conclusion I return to more recent treatment of the psychological diagnosis that complements, strikingly, the essentializing positions of Dawson and his early modern ancestors. If centuries of reporting on this practice have not revealed much culturally specific analysis and conclusion, the exoticizing impulse has remained particularly strong. Maternalized men appear to play a predictable and consistent role in the overall view of cultures of conquest conveniently and consistently turned on their head.

This chapter, while most concerned with the couvade's meaning in the early modern era, contextualizes this curious site of maternal appropriation within

---

[3] Warren Dawson, *The Custom of the Couvade* (Manchester, 1929). The text is also reprinted in Nor Hall's *Broodmales: A Psychological Essay on Men in Childbirth* (Dallas, 1989).

[4] Hilary Klein, "Couvade Syndrome: Male Counterpart to Pregnancy," *International Journal of Psychiatry in Medicine*, 21/1 (1991): pp. 57–69.

discourses from both classical and medieval texts, and follows it through to the seventeenth-century travel narratives of missionaries and explorers. The depiction of the bedridden, newly minted fathers offers up a familiar portrait of otherness and abjection against which the describers and their putative readers may compare and judge their own society. The postpartum father is defined, almost exclusively, by foreignness and anxiety, notions inflected in this case by a departure from gender norms. A father who would indulge in such irrational behavior is described predictably as barbaric, indecipherable, and often comical. Such were the couvade's uses in stories of lands both geographically and culturally far removed from their author's experience. In the early modern period, moreover, this story became ever more immediate as the accounts were, indeed, less fantastical and more observable: explorers could claim to recount what they saw with their own eyes; Brazilians were imported and paraded before their rapt, European spectators and accounts of their bizarre customs preceded them. This chapter investigates the impulse to which Michel de Certeau alludes in the epigraph and which he considers in a similar vein with regard to the sixteenth-century traveler, Jean de Léry: To what extent does the power of the word—story, writing—bear witness to and enact a history of conquest, perpetrated, in these particular examples of couvade, through the norms of gender?

Two pre-Renaissance sources are instructive in establishing the terrain for this discussion: the works of the Greek geographer and historian Strabo (64 BCE–24 CE) and the anonymous *chantefable*, *Aucassin et Nicolette* (thirteenth century). While the direct reception of these sources with respect to the couvade is unclear in the works of the early modern accounts (though Strabo was certainly a general source and model for Renaissance cosmographers), their characterizations of the phenomenon suggest a generalized attitude toward such nonconformist male behavior that serves us well. The retellings of the couvade are suffused with the early modern humanist writer's *modus operandi* as a borrower, an imitator, and a re-inventor: the fingerprints of an enduring fascination and anxiety with the couvade are clear and telling. As Frank Lestringant has observed of the classical resonances in the travel accounts of Thevet, one of the sixteenth-century writers considered in this chapter, "Le lointain dans le temps et le lointain dans l'espace se rejoignent, définissant un commun territoire où la culture humaniste se trouve chez elle, en pays de connaissance" [The distant past and distant lands come together, helping to define a common territory where humanist culture finds a common ground of knowledge].[5]

Postpartum Forefathers

Strabo mentions the custom in his *Geographia*. Embedded in his discourse on the confounding and amoral practices of the Iberians and "their ferocity and bestial insensibility," Strabo relates:

---

[5] Frank Lestringant (ed.), *Le Brésil d'André Thevet: Les Singularités de la France Antarctique* (1557) (Paris, 1997), p. 25.

> For example, these women till the soil, and when they have given birth to a child they put their husbands to bed instead of going to bed themselves and minister to them; and while at work in the fields, oftentimes, they turn aside to some brook, give birth to a child, and bathe and swaddle it.[6]

Denise McCoskey's study of Strabo's *Geography* with regard to women prepares a discussion of how persistently the transgression of gender haunts the European imagination later.[7] Strabo's depiction of women, according to McCloskey, evinces the validation and promotion of Roman imperialism (59); the position of women, she states, "is often used to help 'diagnose' that culture as either barbaric or civilised," all of which is "circumscribed by a particular uneasiness about power and women's autonomy" (61). Though McCoskey's focus is on women, she translates her approach when talking of men and couvade as part of "a formulation that begins to suggest [Strabo's] reliance on inversion as an organising principle of the entire society" (63). Strabo's discussion of the Amazons is characterized as a society in which men were women and women were men, a cautionary world upside down kept consciously and conveniently at the border of the known and unknown:

> Thus, the ancient Greeks made the inverse geographic origins of themselves and the Amazons a key component of their account. So powerful was this paradigm that the Amazon homeland shifted as Greek knowledge of the world increased—precisely so that the Amazons could remain situated at a conceptual border that symbolically elided known/unknown with male/female. (70)

Such is the case in the early modern period, as well as the newly known worlds of the southern hemisphere presented persistently confounding counter-examples to the European imagination. Unsurprisingly, perhaps, in Strabo's account and in those that follow, this de-masculinizing of the exotic male goes hand in hand with parallel attitudes and accounts of the masculinization of their female counterparts: the Amazons, marauding, separatist communities of women with bodies honed for battle and little interest in men beyond what is reproductively necessary. We return to this in our discussion of the seventeenth-century sources in particular.

---

[6] Strabo, *Geographia*, Book III (iv, 17), trans. H.L. Jones (Cambridge, 1969), p. 113.

[7] Denise Eileen McCoskey, "Gender at the Crossroads of Empire: Locating Women in Strabo's *Geography*," in Daniela Dueck, Hugh Lindsay, and Sarah Pothecary (eds), *Strabo's Cultural Geography: The Making of a Kolossourgia* (Cambridge, 2005). For critical geographers, she states, "geography serves as an intellectual or textual procedure by which the world is simultaneously structured and assigned value. In helping to establish and regulate relationships of power, geographic discourses thus parallel other operations of social differentiation" (57).

Before encountering several instances of the couvade as expressed in accounts of the sixteenth- and seventeenth-century voyages of discovery, I propose an exploration of a medieval precedent in the tale of *Aucassin et Nicolette*. This anonymous *chantefable* of the thirteenth century spins the couvade with neo-Rabelaisian humor (replete with food fight) and prepares the discussion of its persistent value as a marker of alterities of race and gender. *Aucassin et Nicolette* is an *ur*-text that, consciously or not, both responds to the classical accounts of Strabo and others that precede it and informs the literary and cultural terrain in which subsequent accounts take root. The couvade scene in this story, though its reception throughout the early modern period is rather unknown, prepares quite perfectly this strange cultural phenomenon played out at the geographic and cultural outposts of barbarism. Anxiety pervades the scene of encounter and the stage is set for subsequent accounts of cultural inscrutability as told through the spectacle of exotic lyings-in.

Aucassin et Nicolette is a story that exploits the couvade motif through the incorporation of a persistently strong woman contrasted throughout with a pathetic, weak male figure whose "prise de conscience" occurs precisely at the moment that he witnesses a father's lying-in. *Aucassin et Nicolette*, as the contrasting lovers' names suggest from the onset, is an unsubtle treatment of the embattled union of opposites, told in the context of a world upside down that must be righted for the lovers' (and society's) eventual satisfaction. Aucassin, the son of an aging local lord, falls desperately in love with Nicolette, an adopted slave girl, newly rebaptized, but clearly unfit for a noble swain, however appropriate his Saracen-sounding name should appear. This is the troubadour's conceit: Aucassin's exotic moniker points to a host of inappropriate behaviors that compromise him severely until he can eventually triumph over them. He plays the whining, incapacitated, and clueless foil to Nicolette's utterly strong and capable heroine.[8] The narrative exploits with constant glee this device of the *monde à l'envers*, the hero in a perpetually compromised state of confusion, while his derring-do damsel navigates the series of trials and exploits with consummate skill and bravery: if Aucassin's primary mode is that of paralysis and lament, Nicolette is, from the start, active and unfazed by tribulation. In this tale of lovers and expected roles turned on their head, it is the spectacle of the couvade that provides the crucial turning point in the story, a defining event that has everything to do with other appearances in the early modern period.

[8] In a telling reversal of poetic tradition, Aucassin is described from toe to head, an indication that he will find his way in the courtly world with difficulty, his reactions and emotions often the opposite or reverse of standard expectations: "Biax estoit et gens et grans et bien tailliés de ganbes et de piés et de cors et de bras; il avoit les caviax blons et menus recercelés et les ex vairs et rians et le face clere et traitice et le nes haut et bien assis" [Handsome, elegant, tall, he had legs, feet, torso, and arms that were well turned out; he had soft, blond ringlets for hair, bright, sparkling eyes, a luminous, refined countenance and a high, well-placed nose.] *Aucassin et Nicolette*, ed. Mario Roques (Paris, 1982), p. 2.

After an agonizing series of tests that culminate (however temporarily) in the reunion of the two lovers, Aucassin and Nicolette flag down a ship and climb on board hoping to find their way home. In a turn of events not unlike those that will beset the beleaguered voyagers in *L'Isle des hermaphrodites* in 1605 (see Chapter 5), a storm picks up, the foreign seas become treacherous, and the ship runs off course and into the port of a strange island: "en haute mer, une tormente leva, grande et mervelleuse, qui les mena de tere en tere, tant qu'il ariverent en une tere estragne et entrerent il port du castel de Torelore" [On the high seas, a storm picked up, large and frightening, that pushed them from one land to the next until they arrived in a foreign place and entered the port of the castle of Torelore] (29–30). Aucassin, increasingly self-possessed and confident in his role as a valiant, heroic male, sets off to visit the king and finds him in a most curious condition:

> [I]l vint el castel; il demande u li rois estoit, et on li dist qu'il gissoit d'enfent. "Et u est don't se femme?" Et on li dist qu'ele est en l'ost et si i avoit mené tox ciax du pais. (30)
>
> [He arrived at the castle. He inquired as to the whereabouts of the king and they told him that he was in childbed. "And so where is his wife?" And they told him that she was in battle and had led all of the inhabitants with her.]

Stupified, Aucassin, sword at his side, charges up to the castle to find the king:

> "Di va! Fau, que fais tu ci?"
> Dist le rois: "Je gis d'un fil;
> quant mes mois sera conplis
> et je sarai bien garis,
> dont irai le messe oir,
> si com mes ancestre fist,
> et me grant guerre esbaudir
> encontre mes anemis;
> nel lairai mie." (30)
>
> ["My word! You fool, what are you doing?"
> Said the king: "I've just had a son;
> when my month is up
> and I'm restored to health
> then I'll go hear a Mass
> just as my ancestors did
> and then return to do battle
> with my enemies;
> I shall not neglect my duties."]

Aucassin's reaction is swift and violent. He slices through the bedclothes of the king, flinging them to the other side of the room. He then picks up a stick and batters the king, almost to death:

> "Ha! Biax sire," fait le rois, "que me demandés vos? Avés vos le sens dervé, qui en me maison me batés?"
>
> "—Par le cuer Diu!" Fait Aucassins, "malvais fix a putain, je vos ocirai, se vos ne m'afiés que ja mais hom en vo tere d'enfant ne gerra." (31)
>
> ["Ah! Dear lord," said the king, "what do you want of me? Are you out of your mind that you should attack me so in my own home?"
>
> "For God's sake!" said Aucassin, "you filthy son of a whore, I will kill you if you will not promise me that never again will a man from your country take to bed after the birth of their child."]

The king consents and Aucassin takes off on his horse, leaving Nicolette in the queen's chambers—as if to indicate the more proper gender assignment upon which Aucassin is insisting. The outraged hero soon finds himself in the midst of the reported battle being waged, much to his continued consternation, not with conventional arms, but with rotten apples, eggs, and cream cheese. His new-found virile comportment is now disastrously inappropriate and he is brought to an exotic form of reason by the king, who explains, "il n'est mie costume que nos entrocions li uns l'autre" [it is not at all our custom to kill each other] (32).

The spectacle of the kingly couvade is a primal drama for Aucassin and a turning point in his chivalric education. Here, he faces all that he might loathe in himself: the effeminized, immobile, and self-absorbed man who allows his wife to rule in what should be his proper domain. Aucassin's violence, even in the context of a highly comical fable, is remarkably robust, marking a transference of his anxieties onto the figure of the king.[9] At the castle of Torelore, Aucassin sees in the king's behavior a personal comportment to be called out and expunged, a loathing predicated on sheer anger or repressed desire (see previous note). Here, lying in childbed, is the old Aucassin, a specter of his former self that incites deep anger and violence. It follows on the heels of another test of his observational

[9] While a development of the psychodynamic drama being rehearsed here is not possible, this scene appears to present a classical case study for Freud's theories of projection and transference, with the protagonist calling out and loathing what he most despises in himself. See Sigmund Freud, "Fragment of an Analysis of a Case of Hysteria ('Dora')," in Peter Gay (ed.), *The Freud Reader*, (New York, 1989), p. 234. An alternative reading here would be of Aucassin's violence to the person who has enacted the life that he *envies*: the King of Torelore presents to him an example of gender fluidity that Aucassin might have embraced, given his boyhood behaviors and proclivities, but can never actualize.

and relational skills, wherein he comes across a beautiful woodland shelter that Nicolette has constructed to entice him, should he pass that way.

> Jure Diu qui ne menti,
> ce par la vient Aucasins
> et il por l'amor de li
> ne s'I repose un petit,
> ja ne sera ses amis,
> n'ele s'amie. (20–21)
>
> [She swears by Holy God
> that if Aucassin comes by there
> and for love of her
> does not rest there awhile
> then never shall he be her lover,
> nor she his.]

Aucassin passes this test: he recognizes the hand of the artist and cannot resist remaining a while in her presence. Aucassin's successful apprehension of his lover's signifying hut, as it were, prepares a similar test of his perception when confronted with the vision of himself in childbed. The violence of his emotions is an invitation for the readers and listeners as well to take such moments of gender transgression for all they are worth. As with the tapestry tableaux of the extreme corporeal violence of Heliogabulus's unsuccessful sex change in the *L'Isle des hermaphrodites* that the bewildered explorers are led to contemplate (see Chapter 5), here again we are given an invitation to decrypt and question. What are the meanings, what is the currency of troubling with one's sex and gender?

If *Aucassin et Nicolette* is a narrative of travel and discovery—both geographic and personal—so can be characterized some of the ensuing accounts of couvade as retold by real-life, early modern explorers. As with the anonymous poet's exotic and entertaining tale of the erstwhile postpartum king, so do a host of other accounts invite our scrutiny for what they tell of reproductive and cultural otherness. *Aucassin et Nicolette* and Rabelais's adventures prepare what are enduring and significant elements in the couvade as we go from fictional "worlds upside down" to "real" ones. That is to say, *their* tales take place in fictional realms where the confusion of gender roles is either didactic or poignantly comical for literary or narrative effect. Aucassin's (and our) "reading" of the couvade scene is a lesson, whether serious or tongue-in-cheek, as to the right ruling of the world by gender as told in the bumbling missteps of its slow-to-enlightenment protagonist. But that is the way things *are* in Torelore, this far-flung foreign land whose protocols and practices around birth—this most significant and fertile of cultural moments—are also turned on their head. Gargantua is born out of his mother's head; his son's birth will also rely on a certain reversal of social practice as he "labors" and nurtures in unconventional ways. Such are the fictional strains and uses of the couvade. It remains to investigate what becomes of such accounts become "fact."

Eyewitnessing Maternal Men across the Seas

Turning to purportedly eyewitness accounts of the couvade from sixteenth- and seventeenth-century French travelers, we find chroniclers whose descriptions of the southern hemisphere lead us to believe that they might truly have found the world on its head. The gendering of the New World is consistently orchestrated so as to portray savage sex roles with regard to birthing as inverted and thus incommensurate with the astonished "discoverer's" norm. Louis Montrose has explored the larger question of the effeminized "savage" in the early modern English context through the example of Sir Walter Ralegh and his exploration of Guiana.[10] His study of the process of "protocolonialist 'othering'" as evidenced in both narrative and graphic depictions of the Americas is deeply informed by questions of gender and power and serves us well here:

> By subsuming and effacing the admired societies of Amerindian men in the metaphorically feminine Other of the land, the English intent to subjugate the indigenous peoples of Guiana can be "naturalized" as the male's mastery of the female. The ideology of gender hierarchy sanctions the Englishmen's collective longing to prove and aggrandize themselves upon the feminine body of the New World, and, at the same time, the emergent hierarchical discourse of colonial exploitation and domination reciprocally confirms that ideology's hegemonic force. (188)

We find complementary evidence in the French accounts of the New World and endeavor to interpret them in the light of what might have helped generate them: overarching colonialist impulses and rhetoric within the specific historical and cultural context in which they are presented. Montrose discusses the specific interests of Queen Elizabeth in this period, whose naming of Virginia was not inconsequential, as well as the competing interests of the Spanish in the colonial enterprise.[11] Here too we remain mindful of the political realities of this period

[10] Louis Montrose, "The Work of Gender in the Discourse of Discovery," in Stephen Greenblatt (ed.), *New World Encounters* (Berkeley, 1993).

[11] The Spanish are depicted as particularly brutal in Ralegh's accounts so as to render English dominion more benevolent: "By the persistent rehearsal of Spanish atrocities against the Indians, the English also tried to turn Spanish precedence to their own advantage. Ralegh could assure himself and his English readers that God had reserved Guiana for England's dominion; and at the same time … he could represent his own imperialistic venture as a holy and humanitarian war of liberation against Spanish oppression." Montrose, "The Work of Gender," p. 193.

for France that motivate these similarly protocolonialist accounts in ways that, interestingly, do not always neatly equate the "savage" with the "other."

We begin with a somewhat more tame and suggestive illustration from Rabelais's contemporary, André Thevet. Thevet was a Franciscan priest, writer, explorer, cartographer, cosmographer to Charles IX, and eventual chaplain to Catherine de Médicis. His work's multiple prefatory dedications by the Pléiade poets of France testify to a highly privileged status in political and literary circles. He made his first trip to the Greek isles and the Levant and the second to Brazil. Unfortunately for him, he became deathly ill on the trip to Brazil and never much left the ship for the 10 weeks he was there. Thevet's writing on this society is based almost entirely on reports of others and observations from his sickbed on the beach, not so far removed from the fictional endeavors of our previous chroniclers—though that may be the point. There is also much in his account that is cribbed from others' writings, making of the *Cosmographie* (and its predecessor, *Les Singularités de la France Antarctique* of 1557) a highly contested conglomeration of texts from multiple sources.[12] Thevet's text, then, relates this concerning the birthing practices of the local indigenous tribe:

> Trois jours durant le Cheroup, ou pere, se tient aupres de sa femme faisant abstinence de toute chair … & mesme ne fait aucune oeuvre, jusques à ce que le nombril de l'enfant soit sec & tombé: de peur (disent-ils) que luy ne l'enfant, ne sa mere n'ayent les trenchees, qu'ils appellent Tekéaip. Il mect aussi par chacun jour, au matin, à midy, & au soir, le pied sur le ventre de sa femme, faisant plusieurs ceremonies presagieuses, comme de petites attrapes faintes à prendre bestes … le tout à fin qu'à l'advenir (disent-ils) l'enfant prenne & tue bestes, oyseaux, & pesche du poisson, avec une infinité d'autres ceremonies superstitieuses qui ne meritent estre recitees. Et si le mary n'y est: le frere de la femme ou son plus proche parent, font tout ce que dessus.[13]
>
> [For three days the "Cheroup," or father, remains at his wife's bedside, abstaining from all meat … and performs no work at all, until the baby's umbilical cord dries and falls off: this done out of fear (so they say) that neither he, nor the child, nor his mother get cramps that they call "Tekéaip." Each day, morning,

[12] See Frank Lestringant's introduction to *Le Brésil d'André Thevet*. The attribution of the work was of no small dispute and prompted, days after its publication, a lawsuit from Mathurin Héret, who claimed to have compiled the accounts of the still ailing Thevet with those of a previous voyager, Villegagnon. Says Lestringant quite succinctly, "Il reste que Thevet publie sous son nom en décembre 1557 le fruit d'une enquête collective et anonyme, à laquelle, en raison de sa maladie prolongée, il n'eu presque aucune part" [And so it is that Thevet publishes under his own name in December of 1557 the fruits of a collective and anonymous effort in which, because of his prolonged illness, he played practically no part.] Lestringant, *Le Brésil d'André Thevet*, p. 21.

[13] André Thevet, *Cosmographie universelle*, vol. II (Paris, 1575), p. 916.

> noon, and night, he puts his foot against his wife's stomach while performing a variety of superstitious rituals such as hanging little animal traps over the child in the hope (so they say) that the child will grow to catch and kill beasts, birds, and fish—this, along with a variety of other superstitious ceremonies not worth telling. And if the husband is not there, the wife's brother or her closest male family member does all of the above.]

While somewhat less dramatic than *Aucassin et Nicolette* or *Gargantua* in its description of thc immobilized father, this spectacle of the postpartum family implies a confounding social universe in which the provider and protector of the family exhibits a cessation of activity. Curiously, Thevet suggests that the father immobilizes himself for fear that *he* (mentioned first) might not experience these postpartum cramps: "de peur (disent-ils) que *luy* ne l'enfant, ne sa mere n'ayent les trenchees [out of fear (so they say) that neither *he*, nor the child, nor his mother get cramps] (my emphasis). He appears to take priority in this birth recovery scenario. The father is completely involved and purposeful in his bonding with both mother and child, performing a physical proximity of exaggerated proportions—at her side, hovering over the child or kneading his wife's stomach with his foot, a display of intense corporeal connection lasting far beyond what might be necessary for, say, compression of the postpartum uterus, as is advised in some gynecological manuals of the period.[14] The account is a fascinating combination of attentiveness to detail as Thevet records the indigenous terminology for gynecological maladies (Tekéiap) and paternalistic dismissiveness regarding the veracity of such accounts ("so they say") and their value ("a variety of other superstitious ceremonies not worth telling"). Thevet's linguistic mastery of their culture gives license to the judgment and censuring of his subject with even greater authority.

Of complementary interest here is the depiction of the mother's labor, which Thevet describes as a venture that takes more or less half a day and is accomplished in remarkable solitude:

> Quand le temps d'enfanter est venu, elles se vont assoir sur une busche de bois platte, laquelle est attachee par dedans aux lattes de la couverture de la maison, & touche à terre, & alors elle jettent quelques cris en leur langaige, assez grands,

---

[14] See, for example, Louise Boursier in her *Observations*, Book I, Chapter XVI and XVII, wherein she advises on the compression of the womb by trussing and various oral remedies, including egg yolks. *Observations diverses sur la stérilité, perte de fruicte, accouchements, et maladies des femmes, et enfants nouveaux naiz*, ed. Françoise Olive (Paris, 1992), pp. 82–3. Laurent Joubert also weighs in on a cure for cramps in a similar vein, advising "que son ventre ne soit un peu pressé, les cuisses croisées pour empêcher le refroidissement et morfondement de la matrice" [that her belly be compressed, and her thighs crossed in order to impede the cooling down or hardening of the womb]. *La Médecine et le régime de santé: des erreurs populaires et propos vulgaires* [1578–79], vol. II, ed. Madeleine Tiollais (Paris, 1997), p. 195.

> disans Akéééli Akaih, ouaih! Qui sont interjections de douleurs communes aux femmes, mesmes quant elles sentent quelque mal: & sont en ce travail environ demy jour (les unes plus les autres moins) sans estre aydees ne secouruës de quelque personne que ce soit. (915)
>
> [When the time of birthing arrives, they go sit on a block of flat wood which is attached to the rafters of their house, reaching down to the ground, and they then let out several rather loud cries in their language, saying "A-kay-lee, A-kay, Oo-ay!," which are the cries of misery common to all women, even those ailing and not in labor: and they remain in this state of labor about half a day (some more some less) without help or succor from any person whatsoever.]

Such observations resonate quite closely with Thevet's description elsewhere in the *Cosmographie* where he resuscitates the myth of the new Amazon community of women who are utterly self-reliant and remarkably valorous and capable in war. The author's blending of myth, conjecture, eyewitness account, and previous explorers' observations serves him well in his portrayal of reversed sex roles. In Chapter 12 of the *Cosmographie*, Thevet is at pains to explain that this mythological sorority vaunted by the Greeks and Romans does *not* inhabit this equatorial region as others may have claimed—no more so than the mermaids or dryads of those fantastical accounts (vol. I, 444a). There is, however, a pair of single-sex islands, Imaugle for the women and Inebile for the men. Thevet assures us he has seen them with his own eyes: "Mais à fin d'oster chacun de debat, & suyvant ce qui en a esté vrayement observé par moy, je deduiray le tout à la verité" [To put a close to this debate, and according to what I actually observed, I will dedicate all of this to the truth] (vol. I, 443a). It appears that something remarkably close to the Amazonian community *does* exist. The women of these islands live separately from their husbands, communing only occasionally for the purposes of procreation and the resettling of their progeny in their proper domains. Thevet cannot resist the Amazonian comparison and his description leaves little room for discernment between the inhabitants of Imaugle and their mythic ancestors he pretends to dismiss:

> Advint aussi, que environ l'an mil cinq cens trentequatre, & quarante & un, ayans leurs ennemis saccagé & pillé la plus part de l'isle où les hommes se tiennent, elles determinerent la guerre contre leurs anciens ennemis pour venger l'injure. Ainsi dresserent elles leur equippage de deux cen batteaux, & mirent bon nombre de filles & de femmes les plus fores qu'elles peurent choisir, en attendant le secours de leurs maris & alliez. (vol. I, 444)
>
> [And it occurred in about 1534 and 1541 that having seen most of the men's island sacked and pillaged, they (the Amazons) determined to wage war against these old enemies and avenge themselves. And so they assembled a fleet of two

> hundred boats and loaded them up with a great number of the strongest girls and women they could find while waiting for the aid of their husbands and friends.]

Clearly these women were not going to wait long. After a long digression on magic and magnetic stones said to be used in the islands, Thevet implores us, "Revenons à noz nouvelles guerrieres d'Imaugle" [So let's get back to our female warriors of Imaugle]:

> Incontinent qu'elles eurent fait descente en la terre de leurs ennemis, qui jamais ne se fussent doubtez de ceste entreprise courageuse de ces femmes, Dieu sçait de quelle fureur ces nouvelles Amazones s'acharnerent sur les pauvres habitans de l'isle de Bazacate, & à les faire mourir cruellement & pauvrement: lesquels ne pouvans resister à ceste tempeste feminine, furent contraints se retirer aux montaignes & grotesques. (vol. I, 445b)
>
> [As soon as they disembarked in the land of their enemy, who were unsuspecting of the courageous nature of these women, God knows with what fury these new Amazons set upon the poor inhabitants of the Island of Bazacate, killing them so pitifully and cruelly. Their victims, unable to defend themselves against this female onslaught, were forced to retreat up into the mountain caves.]

Thevet's indulging of the Amazonian myth is part and parcel of his mosaic-style borrowing from the classical sources that he uses to amplify his accounts, and is entirely resonant with the gender inversion that this new society presents. Montrose speaks of this same gesture in Ralegh's digressions on South American culture and the characterization works in much the same way in the work of Thevet and successive explorers:

> This Amazonian anticulture precisely inverts European norms of political authority, sexual license, marriage and child-rearing practices, and inheritance rules. Such conceptual precision suggests that it was not merely the antiquity and wide diffusion of the idea of the Amazons that compelled Ralegh and his contemporaries to entertain seriously the possibility of their existence. Elizabethan perception and speculation were structured by the cognitive operations of hierarchy and inversion, analogy and antithesis. By the logic of these operations, a conceptual space for reversal and negation was constructed within the world picture of a patriarchal society. Among those figures which might occupy this space were the Amazons. Since they didn't exist, it proved necessary to invent them—or, in the case of the New World, to reinvent them (Montrose 202).

The inscription of this Amazonian anticulture as enhanced by the effeminized men who linger in childbed seems entirely revelant to the French example. One cannot help noting the irony that Thevet is taking observational notes on this inverted culture while languishing in his own metaphorical childbed: his *Singularités* are born(e) out of a protracted, feverish labor of no small proportions!

Brazil's Road to Rouen

If Montrose contextualizes the gendered, protocolonialist rhetoric of Ralegh within the politics of Elizabethan England's struggle for power against Spain, Michael Wintroub's work suggests a parallel set of circumstances in France. In his book, *A Savage Mirror*, he uses the well-documented entrance of Henri II into Rouen in the fall of 1550 as a set-piece for studying the ways in which the performance of the New World embodied the dynamics of power and self-representation in the very decade of Thevet's and his contemporaries' accounts.[15] The staging of this monumentally extravagant entrance includes the participation of actual Brazilians imported for the occasion and featured as representative of France's past and future in world politics. His study of the uses of the New World savage to create a narrative about the glory of France may help to nuance our reception of the curious cases of male maternity that prevail in accounts of French travelers.

The entrance begins with a series of tableaux paraded before the king depicting the glories of both the city of Rouen and of the king himself.[16] Clergy, merchants, tradesmen, lawyers, and military regiments strolled before the king, majestically enthroned in a sumptuously decorated observation box. One after the other, chariots rumbled by, depicting historical triumphs of the mythological past as well as the heroic feats of Henri's campaigns in Boulogne and England. Spoils, captives, and victors are paraded along as casts of hundreds are pressed into service for each "movement" of this living diorama, some of the players culled from the actual regiments—from Normandy, for example—who had recently fought with the king. At the midpoint of this spectacle, the mode of observation then changes: Henri and his entourage of some 300 household officers, gentlemen, and guards descend from their perch and begin the triumphal ride through the town themselves. Here, at this moment that marks the separation between past and future, Henri literally takes to the road again with his gigantic cast of subjects and supporters. He is en route to the final tableau—the Elysian Fields, a utopian, post-battle scene that exalts the renaissance of letters as ushered in by his father, François, whose presence here attaches to them both the reputation of "restaurateur des bons ars & sciences." But to arrive there, they must pass through the dramatically staged spectacle of Brazilian culture that serves as a mediating tableau, negotiating France's bellicose past and, hopefully, pacified future. This interpretive moment is not unlike the scene in which Aucassin comes upon several significant tableaux himself in the

15 Michael Wintroub, *A Savage Mirror: Power, Identity, and Knowledge in Early Modern France* (Stanford, 2006).

16 I rely here on the facsimile version of the entrance with introduction by Margaret M. McGowan, *L'Entrée de Henri II, Rouen 1550* (Amsterdam, 1974).

chantefable, most notably the drama of the king's couvade. The narrative trail, as it were, is rich and worth investigating for what it portends for royal men and specifically, in the case of Henri II, who embody this *renaissance*. Significant as well, perhaps, is the specter of violence that accompanies these moments of recognition, change, and rebirth. The delivery of this new society is not without its transformational pain.

At this moment of transition, Henri stops along the banks of the Seine and gazes upon a scene of remarkable artistry and industry—an entire Brazilian village populated in part by authentic indigenous people imported for the occasion:

> Le long de la place se demenoient ca & la, jusques au nombre de trois centz hommes tous nudz … sans aucunement couvrir la partie que nature commande, ilz estoient faconnez & equipez, en la mode des sauvages de l'amerique … du nombre desquelz il y en avoit bien cinquante naturelz sauvages, freschement aportez du pays … Le surplus de la compagnie, ayant frequente le pays, parloit autant bien le langage, & exprimoit si nayfvement les gestes & facons de faire des sauvages, comme s'ilz fussent natifz du mesmes pays.[17]
>
> [Throughout the scene were running about, here and there, up to 300 men, all naked … without even covering the parts that nature commands they were made up and equipped in the style of American savages of whom there were 50 real savages, freshly imported from their country … The remainder of the cast, having visited the country, spoke the language rather well and performed the gestures and ways of the savages so naturally as to be taken for natives of that same country.]

The Brazilians, real and simulated, gambol about chasing after imported monkeys and exotic birds, dancing, harvesting wood (painted red to resemble Brazilian species), fishing, and, eventually, waging a battle with a neighboring, rival tribe. Arrows fly, men and women dance and flee, a general chaos of both pacific and violent interactions occurs simultaneously as the remarkable discoveries of the New World are trotted out for the Old. Both the written and visual narrations of this *son et lumière*-like spectacle (*avant la lettre*) suggest a vertiginous, multi-layered tableau of stunning proportions (see Figure 6.1). The woodcut that accompanies the account (*Figure des Brisilians*) captures at least the fantasy of Henri's view with a totalized, simultaneous view of this culture of conquest and commerce. At once Edenic and apocalyptic (and many practical, present-day things in between), the tableau presents couples and groups of people strolling or dancing peacefully in carefree leisure; hunters and gatherers going about their daily routines for finding sustenance; loggers and traders transporting goods to ships; and multiple scenes of violent encounter, bows drawn, with both the upper left and right of the

[17] The McGowan facsimile edition includes no pagination. This description is found immediately after the woodcut "Figure des Brisilians." between folios H and K.

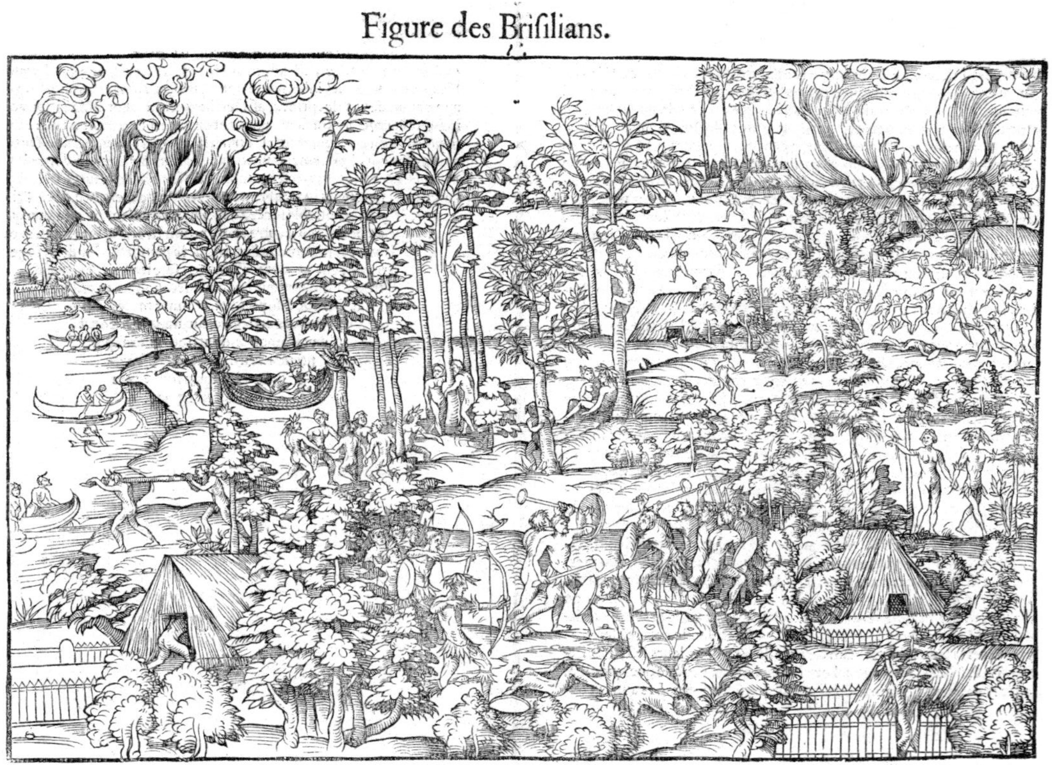

Figure 6.1 *Figure des Brisilians, Cest la deduction du sumptueux ordre, plaisantz spectacles et magnifiques theatres dresses, et exhibes par les citoiens de Rouen...* (1551) [Typ 515 51.272]. Courtesy of Houghton Library, Harvard University.

visual field framed by flames and plumes of smoke, the perpetual fiery background to their day-to-day existence.

Wintroub's unpacking of this spectacle places the tableau of the Brazilians in the context of France's particular political, military, and cultural moment, and, as such, the reading is inflected in somewhat unexpected ways. His very convincing reading of this event, which he characterizes as "civilizing the savage and making a king" (39), interprets the savage as both foil for and representative of the contemporary Frenchman. His interpretation of the uses of Hercules in the tableau just after the Brazilian village scene encapsulates this well:

> Half man and half god, emblem of savagery as well as of civilization, Hercules was known for his heroic strength as well as for his powers of eloquence. Like the Brazilians, he stood for—and mediated between—contrasting ideals of what it meant to be an elite in early modern France ... Both the Brazilians and Hercules embodied values central to the identity of France's nobility, values such as bravery, strength, and skill in battle ... Both were considered to be barbarians who needed to be civilized. (42)

As such, the simulated war was about at least three things: honoring Henri's military prowess; mimicking defeat of the Portuguese in the Atlantic theater; and de-barbarizing the French in contrast to the Italians. A number of contemporary issues and anxieties are therefore collapsed into this complicated tableau wherein questions of national identity and aspiration are trotted out and promoted. As Wintroub suggests, this is the theatrical version of Du Bellay's *Défense et Illustration de la Langue Française*, a realization of France's stature that can rival the European counterparts in battles for land and for letters (42). The French spectator watches as the savage warriors meld into a version of civility with Orpheus and his lyre strumming their passage into the Elysian Fields. The range of meanings attached to this savage are familiar, as Montaigne's observations on cannibals from just this region of the New World decades later still remind us. They are at once violent in their ritualistic cannibalism; noble in their relative purposefulness and justification ("Je pense qu'il y a plus de barbarie à manger un homme vivant qu'à le manger mort" [I think that there is more barbarity in eating a man alive than in eating him dead]); and equal to our cultural self-glorifying mission as witnessed in the sophistication of their poetry ("Or j'ay assez de commerce avec la poësie pour juger cecy, que non seulement il n'y a rien de barbarie en cette imagination, mais qu'elle est tout à fait Anacreontique" [Now I am familiar enough with poetry to be a judge of this: not only is there nothing barbarous in this fancy, but it is altogether Anacreontic.][18] As betrayed in Montaigne's characteristically multivalent and perpetually revised essays and as played out in the agendas evident in the

[18] Michel de Montaigne, *Oeuvres complètes*, ed. Albert Thibaudet and Maurice Rat (Paris, 1962), pp. 207, 212. Translation: *The Complete Works of Montaigne*, Donald M. Frame (Stanford, 1976), pp. 155, 158.

representations, performed, engraved, and written of staged encounters such as the entry of Henri II into Rouen, the currency of the Brazilian savage is vast yet purposeful. I look therefore to subsequent representations of the exotic postpartum male as perhaps further indicative of this interface in which certain markers of exoticism and gender define the terrain with abiding consistency.[19] Incivility, backwardness, and infantile superstition so prevalent in his narratives are mapped onto gender in the birth process, a performance of effeminized manhood—and hyper-masculine femininity—that becomes only more elaborated in the chroniclers that we turn to briefly now.[20]

Couvade and Control of the New World Body

Antoine Biet, a French priest, explorer, and early colonizer, traveled to French Guiana in 1652 and related his observations a decade later in *Voyage de la France équinoxiale en l'isle de Cayenne*. He was one of two priests to survive the hardships during his 15-month stay in the region and published his account in three volumes. The relevant passage, which I quote at length for the number of threads from previous accounts that it incorporates, is a follows:

> Quand la femme mariée reconnoist qu'elle est enceinte, elle se declare à son mary, qui fait alors beaucoup de choses superstitieuses, craignant que l'enfant qu'elle porte ne perisse. Il s'abstient de manger de plusieurs choses; il fait une penitence étroite; il craint de toucher les gros poisons, comme le Lamantin, la Tortuë & semblables. Aussi-tost que la femme est accouchée, ce qu'elle fait avec grande facilité, à cause du grand exercice qu'elles font, & qu'elles ne sont pressées d'aucun vestement; elles se font & à leurs enfans, ce que les Sages-femmes ont accoustumé de faire, n'y en ayant point dans ces païs. Elles se levent sur l'heure, prenant l'enfant entre leurs bras, & se vont laver & luy aussi, dans la Riviere prochaine. Le mary pend son lit au plus haut de la Case, s'y va coucher; & fait l'accouchée six semaines, & au lieu de faire servir sa femme qui ne garde point le lict, elle le sert luy-mesme durant tout ce temps-là, pendant lequel il ne se leve que pour aller à ses necessitez. Quand il passe au milieu de tous ses cohabitans, il ne les regarde pas, ne levant pas les yeux. Il

[19] See also Frank Lestringant's *Cannibals: The Discovery and Representation of the Cannibal from Columbus to Jules Verne*, trans. Rosemary Morris (Berkeley, 1997), specifically Chapter 5 on the complexity of Montaigne's amalgam of views and sources on the cannibal in mid-sixteenth-century nascent French ethnography.

[20] If Thevet has been roundly criticized for the errors and presumptions in his travelogs regarding this "bête brute, sans foi, sans loi, sans religion, sans civilité aucune," it appears some small revenge was meted out early on: while languishing feverishly in his cot, he was seized upon by some local "savage thieves," who left him stark naked, a state he bemoaned and condemned repeatedly in his sour descriptions of their brethren. See Thevet's *Singularitez de la France antarctique* (Paris, 1558), p. 51.

> jeusne étroitement pendant ces six semaines, ne mangeant que fort peu, d'où vient que quand sa couche est faite, il se leve maigre comme une squelette.[21]
>
> [When the wife realizes that she is pregnant, she announces this to her husband, who then begins doing all manner of superstitious things, fearing for the health of the child. He abstains from eating certain things; his life is one of strict penitence; he fears touching large fish, such as manatees, tortoises, and the like. As soon as the wife gives birth, which she does with great ease because of the great work that these women do and because they wear no clothing, she does for herself what [in our society] is accomplished by midwives of which there are none here. The women get up right away, taking the child in their arms and go to wash both themselves and the child in the nearest river. The husband hangs his bed high up in the hut and takes to childbed for six weeks, and, instead of serving his wife who has now left her bed, it is she who serves him the whole time, during which he never gets up except to go to relieve himself. When he passes among his neighbors, he does not look at them and does not raise his eyes. He goes on a strict fast during these six weeks, eating extremely little so that by the time he gets up he is as thin as a skeleton.]

The behavior here is one classed as superstitious, irrational, and vaguely comical. The women give birth effortlessly and the men, as if by compensation, suffer all the more agony in their stead. Again, there is a highly performative caste to this ritual: the husband both goes to bed ("s'y va coucher") and plays the role of the postpartum mother ("fait l'accouchée") for six weeks. Here we sense shades of the grieving Gargantua after his Herculean labor. As in the accounts that we witnessed in Thevet, these savage women are fit for birthing because of their labor in the fields and also, strangely, by dint of their nakedness; these women have no need of midwives; in fact, they turn back to their very own labor room and perform such functions for their newly overcome husbands.[22]

As we return to the question of comparative labors, my investigation is further propelled by the work of Jennifer Morgan, whose work on the nexus of reproduction, racism, and economics puts labor of several sorts at the center of her inquiry. In *Laboring Women*, Morgan takes up the accounts of "exotic" civilizations under increasingly European control as key to the conflation of sexual identity and the development of racialist ideology:

[21] Antoine Biet, *Voyage de la France équinoxiale en lisle de Cayenne, entrepris par les François en l'année* MDCLII–1664 (Paris, 1664), pp. 389–90.

[22] The presumption of the painless child labor of women less civilized than the French appears frequently in medical and popular literature. Guillaume Bouchet's *Serées*, for example (another precursor to *Les Caquets de l'accouchée* to be discussed in my conclusion), includes a lengthy treatment of such hearty heathen women. See Guillaume Bouchet, *Les Serées* (1584, 1597, 1598), ed. C.E. Roybet (Paris, 1872), vol. 4, pp. 51–3.

> The willingness to exploit African women's labor became intimately tied to ideas about reproduction. For European travelers … the enslavement of African laborers required a sense of moral and social distance over those they would enslave. They acquired that distance in part through manipulating symbolic representations of African women's sexuality. European men gradually brought African women into focus—women whose pain-free reproduction (at least to European men) indicated that they did not descend from Eve and who illustrated their proclivity for hard work through their ability to simultaneously till the soil and birth a child. Such imaginary women suggested an immutable difference between Africans and Europeans, a difference ultimately codified as race.[23]

I extend here the discussion to similarly racist imaginings about the men who supported these marvelously insentient Brazilian women who were so conveniently freed to return to work. I propose that the accounts of the couvade in the early modern period might be similarly intentional narratives, driven by agendas that appropriate their subjects, both literally and ideologically, into a New World order. I propose that the practice of the couvade, ripe as it is with such comic, dramatic, and exoticizing potential, is pressed into service in various texts of the era of discovery to link foreign cultures in a familiar web of abjection: a host of barbaric societies tellingly bereft of the civilizing hand of the world right side up.

Jean-Baptiste Du Tertre, was a Dominican missionary to the Antilles traveling at the same time and recording his observations in *Histoire générale des isles de S. Christophe*. If the Eurocentrism of the previous accounts resides principally in the surrounding discourse in which the ritual is embedded (the casting of the "bêtes brutes"), Du Tertre's tale is interlarded with a great deal of headscratching:

> Une de leur sottise qui me choque davantage, est cette superstition que les hommes pratiquent à la naissance des enfans. Les femmes enfantent avec peu de douleur … Et tant s'en faut, qu'elles fassent les symagrées des femmes de l'Europe, l'enfant n'est pas plustost au monde, qu'apres l'avoir lavé & mis dans son petit lict de coton, elles travaillent dans la Case, comme si rien ne s'estoit passé en leur endroit, & comme si le mal de la femme avoit passé jusqu'au mary, il commence à se plaindre & à jetter les hauts cris, de mesme que si on luiy avoit arraché l'enfant du ventre par pieces & par morceaux.
>
> Cependant, on se met en peine de le solliciter: on luy pend promptement un lict au haut de la Case, & là on le visite comme malade; mais on luy fait faire une diette qui gueriroit des gouttes & de la grosse verolle, les plus replets hommes de France. Pour moy, je m'estonne comme ils peuvent tant jeusner sans mourir; car ils passent quelquefois les cinq premiers jours, sans boire ny manger aucune

---

[23] Jennifer Morgan, *Laboring Women: Reproduction and Gender in New World Slavery* (Philadelphia, 2004), pp. 7–8.

> chose, & jusqu'au dixieme ils ne font que boire du ouycou, qui peut autant nourrir que de la bierre.
>
> Les quarante jours expirez, ils invitent leurs parens & meilleurs amis, lesquels estant arrivez auparavant que de se mettre à manger, vous découpent la peau de ce pauvre miserable avec des dents d'Acouty, & tirent du sang de toutes les parties de son corps, en sorte que d'un malade par pure imagination, ils en font bien souvent un malade réel.[24]
>
> [One of their stupidities that shocked me even more is this superstition that the men practice upon the birth of their children. The women give birth painlessly … so much so that they make fools out of European women, the child is barely born and these mothers have washed it and put it in its little cotton bed and they are back at work in the hut as if nothing had just happened and as if the pain of their condition had passed along to their husband, who sets to complaining and crying out loudly as though one had just torn a child out of his belly by bits and pieces.
>
> Great pains are taken to attend to him: a bed is set up promptly in the hut and he is visited like a sick person; they prepare for him a diet that would cure even the most corpulent of Frenchmen of his gout or syphilis. Me, I'm astonished that they can fast like that and not die, for they sometimes spend the first five days without eating or drinking a thing and then up to the tenth they drink only *ouycou* (a local brew) that can't nourish one much better than beer.
>
> The forty days passed, they invite their family and closest friends … who then cut the skin of this miserable man with the teeth of an *acouty* (hare-like animal) and draw blood from all parts of his body such that this imaginary invalid often becomes a real one.]

While the encounter here pretends to no little comic effect—Du Tertre, the consummate Frenchman, decrying the lack of good food and drink while at the same time hinting at the effects of excess (gout and syphilis)—the observations he makes are a classic embodiment (dare we say) of a racialized, neocolonialist discourse that marks otherness as aberrant and risible and "sameness" as the White, European norm into which all appetites, as it were, must conform. The "sottises" and "superstitions" collide predictably and, indeed, necessarily with the author's unquestionably rational experience of himself. Jim Perkinson's work on the fraught encounters between Black and White within contemporary American culture are particularly relevant. His essay "The Body of White Space," in his words, "demystifies White male embodiment as a privilege of givenness," whose forms, he suggests, operate as follows:

---

[24] Jean-Baptiste Du Tertre, *Histoire générale des isles de S. Christophe, de la Guadeloupe, de la Martinique et autres dans l'Amérique* (Paris, 1654), pp. 412–14.

> They tend to encode technologies of normativity that do not require the work of conscious performance. They constitute an unproblematic physicality in the body politic. They navigate social space—both public and private—unobstructed, un(re)marked … It is this body that stands as the hegemonic body par excellence. Its particular constellation of meanings … are produced and reproduced in discourses that are not simply verbal. Indeed, I will claim that a large part of this body's social inscription is accomplished in and by its production and occupation of certain spaces in a normative "realization" of quite particular protocols.[25]

Perkinson's theorizing of hegemonic constructs as physically charged expressions that are produced, reproduced, and inscribed is particularly apt to the racialization of the New World accounts of exotic men's experience of childbirth that we observe here. If, as he says, the White, male position does not "require" conscious performance, by contrast, the primitive, indigenous population is, to reverse Perkinson's terminology, utterly *abnormal*, *problematically* physical, *obstructive*, and keenly, comically *remarkable*.[26] Interestingly, Perkinson takes up the ritualized, performative practices of non-American, non-European culture—in his instance spirit possession in West Africa—and valorizes this experience as a "thickly textured set of bodily enactments," articulated in highly specific ways that give "dramatic currency to the value and experience of plurality" (176). This, according to Perkinson, stands in marked contrast to the enactments of White middle-class cultures whose manifestations valorize homogeneity: "White embodiment … historically, has been more about the meeting of norms, quietly fitting in, not causing a spectacle. It has been constituted in a gaze that solicits conformity, not subversive stylizations of individuality" (185). Du Tertre's account of the couvade ends in dramatic misery for these inscrutable beings, their bodies slashed by animal teeth and, as he describes later in his account, finally smeared with a chili-pepper paste that all but literally sets them aflame. If Perkinson's accounts grapple with the more contemporary spectacle of Rodney King and the American context of terrorizing, aberrant bodies, his discourse is not unsuited to the "flaming" specter of the postpartum tribesmen. Inexplicable, unassimilable, and consciously so, these laboring men are inscribed into a cultural (and, of course, theological—these are all Catholic missionaries, to be sure) construct that bestows invisible yet omnipresent privilege and power to the inscriber and subjection to the extravagantly savage other.

---

[25] Jim Perkinson, "The Body of White Space: Beyond Stiff Voices, Flaccid Feelings, and Silent Cells," in Nancy Tuana, William Cowling, Maurice Hamington, Greg Johnson, and Terrance MacMullan (eds), *Revealing Male Bodies* (Bloomington, 2002), p. 174.

[26] It is perhaps ironic that one of the most remarkable facets of "savage" childbirth is the relative ease of childbirth that we have already discussed: remarkable because it is seemingly *unremarkable* to the birthers themselves.

Postmortem on Postpartum

Responding to Thevet's infamous phrase regarding his savage subjects as "sans foi, sans loi, sans religion, sans civilité aucune," Janet Whatley writes: "This list of privatives was already a commonplace in early descriptions of the Indian: he is culturally naked; or, to use a favorite metaphor of the time, he and his New World are a *tabula rasa* waiting to receive European inscription."[27] Indeed. The copious dedicatory epistles to André Thevet for his *Cosmographie* by the illustrious poets in Hebrew, Greek, Latin, and French extol him as imbued with the spirit and courage of the ancients, his experience and certainly his descriptive capacity heavily predetermined by their precedent:

> Comme Ulysse eschappé de cent mille dangers,
> De ce qu'il a conquis sur les bords estrangers
> Un eternel trophée il plante sur noz rives:
> Rapportant, non l'honneur d'un peuple surmonté
> Non le riche butin d'un barbare dompté,
> Mais de tout l'univers les despouilles captives. (Thevet, *Cosmologie* e ii verso)
>
> [Like Ulysses who escaped from a hundred thousand dangers
> From those conquered on foreign shores
> An eternal trophy he plants on our banks:
> Bringing back, not the honor of this conquered people,
> Nor the rich booty of a vanquished savage,
> But the captured skins of the entire universe.]

It is into this vision of conquest and acquisition that Thevet and his fellow chroniclers inscribe their mission, a cultural pillaging, as it were, that is fed by foreign bodies that perform in indecipherable ways. Du Bellay suggests that Thevet moves beyond the specific booty of his particular voyage and glorifies the entire project of colonialization, indeed globally, "Mais de tout l'univers les despouilles captives." To encounter the giant tomes of Thevet's *Cosmographie* as a physical object, a "European inscription" of impressive heft, is to witness a "dépouille" of no small consequence: the fact that printing at this age is not so

---

[27] Janet Whatley, "Savage Hierarchies: French Catholic Observers of the New World," *Sixteenth Century Journal*, 1/3 (1986): p. 321. See also Wintroub on the texture of privation that pervades these narratives. Comparing Thevet's account to that of Pero de Magalhaes de Gandavo regarding the same population, he relates: "A strange balance of *withouts* characterized them: they were without kings, but they were also without masters; they were without clothes, but they were also without the artifices of fashionability; they were without laws and, indeed, without writing, but they were also without those affectations which could cloud a more immediate apprehension of truth." Wintroub, *Savage Mirror*, p. 100.

far removed from vellum or actual animal skins only adds to the poignancy of this connection of bodies and bodies of writing. Jean Dorat, the mentor to several of the Pléiade poets who also praises Thevet, makes glorious comparisons as well: "Et nunc Jason, nunc vagus Hercules; Telluris oras eruit ultiimas."[28] Thevet is seen as the literary issue, as it were, of Jason and Hercules, an argonaut and a laborer whose legendary exploits infuse past, present, and future with their example.[29] One can translate Dorat's Latin in two ways: "Now Jason, now wandering Hercules has brought to light—or destroyed—the farthest shores of the Earth." Thevet is inscribed firmly into their example that goes on for several lengthy pages comparing him most favorably. Such encomium begs the question of one's capacity to see what one is encountering; of shedding preconception and classical conditioning, and getting outside one's subjectivity—a subjectivity highly determined by book learning and not so much by experience. But is not the adventure of landing on the shores of Brazil or the Antilles, the very definition of extra-literary exploration and discovery? Perhaps not. For Thevet, Biet, and Du Tertre, encounters with exotic men and their strange practices appears more about subsuming their upside-down world into a preconditioned, classically prepared vision of life below the equator as literally turned on its head. Racism is mapped onto received notions of gender—Amazons will be Amazons; wouldn't it be just like their irrationally, savage, male partners to take to childbed and scream as though their offspring were being torn in pieces from their bellies? As Jennifer Morgan implies, a savage woman, so physically hardened that her child labor barely interferes with her field labor, is a convenient thing. Likewise, a ritually mollified and confused man writhing in the childbed and attended to by his Amazonian wife is all the more risible and in need of civilizing.

The couvade phenomenon is one that has been recorded for thousands of years: as mentioned, the Greek geographer Strabo, like Thevet, more steeped in books than in boats writing at the beginning of the Common Era, described this curious practice among the exotic and barbaric Iberians. There is also an expansive literature concerning the couvade among social scientists today, where it is discussed as a syndrome of somatic anxiety, pseudo-sibling rivalry, statement of paternity, ambivalence about paternity, and parturition envy (in psychological literature), and an affirming rite of passage, bonding, paternal imprinting, and communal celebration (among anthropologists). A recent literature review of the couvade phenomenon in the *Journal of Reproductive and Infant Psychology* is telling in what it betrays of the persistence of Eurocentric

---

[28] See the front matter in Thevet's *Cosmographie* (unpaginated): Joachim du Bellay, "AVTRE SONNET DV MESME AVTHEVR"; Jean Dorat, "IN A. THEVETI COSMOGRAPHICA. ODE. Io. Aurati Poëtae Regii."

[29] We remember here as well the pivotal role of Hercules as transitional figure in the *entrée* of Henri II into Rouen.

bias with regard to the spectacle of men suffering in childbirth.[30] Curiously, the phenomenon, explored here in mainly psychological terms, is re-appropriated into "developed" cultures, though the rhetoric is somewhat more veiled. The abstract begins by stating, "The Couvade syndrome is a global phenomenon occurring in industrialised countries around the world and has a wide international variance" (173). The conclusion begins with the same statement, slightly recast: "The Couvade syndrome is a global phenomenon occurring in developed countries" (187). In this contemporary analysis the study of the couvade has shifted its focus to the purview of "industrialised" and "developed" societies and one might wonder why. The psychodynamic complexity is ever more elaborated with a range of issues that complement those outlined above, including work on hormonal responsiveness in men (180), the fetus as rival (182), a response to marginalization of men during pregnancy and childbirth (183), the development crisis attending to the transition to fatherhood (184), and role preparation (185). Interestingly, within the population groups that were studied, the authors found compelling evidence to suggest that ethnicity played a consistently significant role:

> Ethnicity is one demographic factor whose relationship with the syndrome appears to be consistent. Anthropological studies of three societies by Munroe and Munroe (1971) and Monroe et al (1973) found that Black Caribbean males reported greater number and frequency of symptoms of the syndrome compared to a Caucasian American sample. Similarly Davis (1978) and Clinton (1986) also confirmed a higher incidence of the syndrome among ethnic minorities and black men in the United States. (176)

It appears that the phenomenon remains racialized in revealing ways, though the characterizations change according to the theory that has evolved to explain it. As the tools of analysis move into the complexities of psychodynamic impulses and dramas, the focus shifts (necessarily?) to industrialized and developed populations. Within these modern case studies, however, it is perhaps telling that the most robust instances of such inscrutable masculinity occur within the very societies that first piqued the "civilized" European imagination: Du Tertre was remarking on the very ancestors of these pre-migration minorities 400 years ago. Understanding the couvade, or at least unpacking its inscrutability, must necessarily be nourished by a self-awareness with regard to the exoticizing ancestors I have treated here. This chapter has attempted to explore the instances of men suffering in childbed in ways that shows rather remarkable consistency in approach over time and only suggests, finally, the history of European hegemony embedded in both fiction and eyewitness accounts that

---

[30] Arthur Brennan, Susan Ayers, Hafez Ahmed, and Sylvie Marshall-Lucette, "A Critical Review of the Couvade Syndrome: The Pregnant Male," *Journal of Reproductive and Infant Psychology*, 25/3 (2007): pp. 173–89.

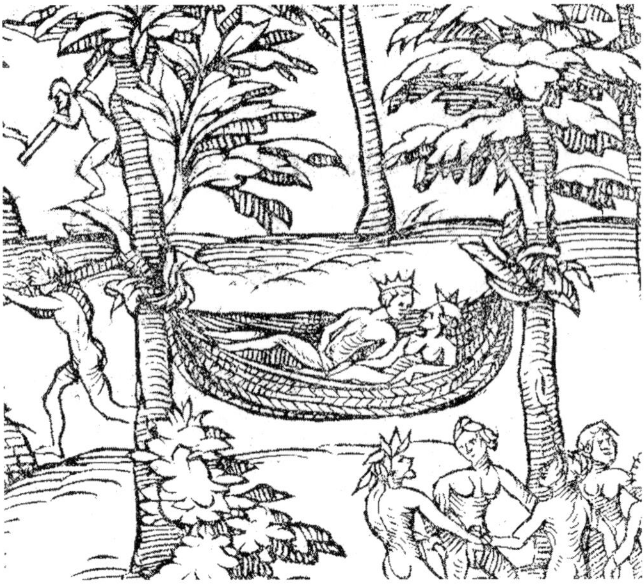

Figure 6.2 Detail, *Figure des Brisilians, Cest la deduction du sumptueux ordre, plaisantz spectacles et magnifiques theatres dresses, et exhibes par les citoiens de Rouen...* (1551) [Typ 515 51.272]. Courtesy of Houghton Library, Harvard University.

deserves more comprehensive, indeed perhaps more generous reception and decoding.

In the pitched battle between colonizer and colonized, one wonders of the possibility for a more complex view of the couvade and its retelling, one that might throw into question the binary imperative into which the "world upside down" of these texts can pull us. Is not part of the appeal of the story of Aucassin and Nicolette the poignancy and iconoclastic glee with which they deny their prescribed roles? Homi Bahbha's admonition to the now postcolonial enterprise is perhaps instructive:

> It must be our aim not to deny or disavow masculinity, but to disturb its manifest destiny—to draw attention to it as a prosthetic reality—a "prefixing" of the rules of gender and sexuality; an appendix or addition, that willy-nilly, supplements and suspends a "lack-in-being." A revisioning, a de-bifurcating of the gendered code here might prove helpful for our past and future.[31]

[31] Homi Bhabha, "Are You a Man or a Mouse?" in Maurice Berger, Brian Wallis, and Simon Watson (eds), *Constructing Masculinity* (New York, 1995), p. 57.

I return to the spectacular woodcut from the printed account of Henri II's entry into Rouen (Figure 6.2), this scene of chaotic activity that so encapsulates France's many agendas in the lands down under. Amidst the industrious loggers, the warring tribesmen, the panicking masses, and the dancing, carefree revelers, there is a vision of domestic tenderness that is arresting. In the center left portion of the tableau, not so very far from the boats arriving to load wood to be shipped back to Europe, is what appears to be a royal couple in bed, swinging in a hammock and clearly engaged in some exchange. It is not, to our eye, immediately identifiable as a childbed—though there does appear to be something strapped to the tree above their heads that could easily resemble a swaddled infant; but the pose, particularly given the rather European-inspired crowns, does suggest the likes of a reconstructed Aucassin and Nicolette. For all the crudity of the medium and the compactness of these multiple scenes of Brazilian life, the image is remarkable in its conveyance of tenderness. The couple's heads are turned to each other, and they are naked but for their royal headgear. It suggests, to a reader of Thevet, something akin to his reporting of the attentive new father compressing his wife's postpartum belly as she recovers from childbirth. Thevet does talk of hanging traps over the bed such as those perhaps sketched in one or the other of the trees to which the hammock is tied, which is to say that there may be evidence in our readings and our apprehension of these accounts that are instructive in positive ways—readings of societies that live in their gender roles, and specifically in their birthing bodies, in ways that are more generous. To be sure, this chaotic scene can be interpreted in the context of a truly bifurcated universe of a lost Eden or impending Apocalypse, a harbinger of the chaos into which France will soon plunge in the latter half of the sixteenth century. But this tender, cocooned royal couple may then still be read as a vision of living outside of the familiar gendered universe and within a vision of more capacious, shared participation in the propagation of its inhabitants. And yet indeed, the spectacle of the couvade for Thevet and those who encountered and recounted after him, was a phenomenon that presented a vision of manhood incommensurate with patriarchal, colonizing Europeans. To deride it was, per force, to exalt a version of the gendered world whose powerful hegemonic discourse went hand in hand with the bloodshed to follow, both home and abroad.

Postpartum

This investigation of the birthing body—its currency, its power, its multiple meanings across genres and gender—began in Chapter 1 by examining the curious case of *Les Caquets de l'accouchée*, penned by an ailing scribe whose condition so mirrors the state of the postpartum mother that he refers to his text as an afterbirth. Here, in what may serve as an epilogue to my own particular retellings of a number of early modern accounts, conventional and otherwise, I invoke one last example from the sixteenth century whose conceit and content are similar to *Les Caquets* and remind us fairly concisely of the range of birthing issues that attend to both the powerful lived experience of generation and to its metaphors for men and women who mined it for literary ends. *Les Serées* by Guillaume Bouchet is a series of "après-dînées," or after-dinner conversations among a fictional, literate, provincial *côterie* whose discussions focus in each session on a specific topic.[1] The three volumes, published successively in 1584, 1597, and 1598, while structured more tightly in a thematic sense than *Les Caquets*, say less about the tellers and attendants; as with the seventeenth-century work, however, one has the impression of a vast gathering of men and women crowding into whatever room could accommodate them as the interlocutors vied for attention through displays of humor and erudition. The narrative is interspersed constantly with "un de la serée a dit," "un autre de la serée leur dit" ["one at the soirée said," "another at the soirée said to them"], with the women, either as hostesses or as interested or implicated parties in the discussions, weighing in from time to time. One impertinent critic of learned women stops short his intervention "de peur d'offenser les femmes, mesme celle qui estoient en ceste Seree, des plus savantes, doctes, bien disantes, avec cela des plus honestes, sages & pudiques qu'on eust peu trouver" [for fear of offending women, particularly those who were at this Soirée, the most learned, wise, and articulate, in addition to being of the

[1] See Hope Glidden, *The Storyteller as Humanist:* The Serées *of Guillaume Bouchet* (Lexington, KY, 1981). Glidden treats the work as one penned for the merchant class of Poitiers (Bouchet had been elected to the mostly honorary position of what might be the equivalent of the president of the local chamber of commerce), a text whose subjects and conversational style witnesses and promotes, to some degree, learned citizenship and erudition. See also André Janier's *Les "Serées," 1584, 1597, 1598, du librairie-imprimeur Guillaume Bouchet (1514–1594)* (Paris, 2006), an exhaustive concordance of the work that serves as an invaluable index for the subjects and their early modern context.

highest integrity, wisdom, and modesty that one could have found].[2] Several of the after-dinner topics lead the conversationalists into realms germane to the birthing body, namely: "Des Femmes, & des Filles" [Of Women and Girls] (third evening); "Des nouvellement mariez & mariees" [Of newly married men and women] (fifth evening); "Des Femmes grosses d'enfans." [Of Women great with child] (22nd evening); "Des Accouchees" [Of Newly-delivered Women] (23rd evening); and "Des Nourrices" [Of Wet Nurses] (24th evening). The opening to the evening dedicated to the pregnant woman is particularly telling and appropriate with regard to the trajectories of both *Les Serées* and *Birthing Bodies*:

> Nous fusmes soupper d'aventure en trois maisons l'une apres l'autre, où nous trouvasmes les Dames du logis en diverse disposition. La premiere estoit grosse: & c'est ceste Seree icy, où il ne fut parlé que des femmes grosses … La seconde estoit en couche, & la Seree fut des femmes qui sont en gesine. La tierce estoit nourrice, & on ne traicta aussi que des femmes qui allaictent leurs enfans. Car tout ce qui se presentoit à nos yeux, ou qu'on entendoit dire, nous servoit de matiere & de livre. Valoit-il pas mieux en ces Serees & convives faire un entremets de choses utiles & profitables, avec une saulse de propos joyeux & recreatifs, que durant le banquet avoir un cruel spectacle de gladiateurs, qui de leur sang & leur cervelle gastoient les habillemens, tachoient les nappes, polluoient les viandes, & remblissoient les coupes? Ne dit pas le Poëte:
>
> Celuy qui le profit & le plaisir assemble,
> Meslangeant dextrement les deux en ses escrits,
> Enseigne & resjouit des lisans les esprits,
> Gaigne le prix d'honneur de tous poincts, ce me semble. (vol. 3, pp. 277–8)
>
> [We went to dine by chance in three houses, one after the other, where we found the Ladies of the house in various conditions. The first was pregnant and this was the Soirée where we spoke only of pregnant women … The second (hostess) was in childbed and this Soirée was about women in labor. The third (hostess) was a wet nurse and there we spoke exclusively of women who were nursing their children. Therefore all that was presented to our eyes and all that we heard tell, provided us with material for our book. Is it not better in these Soirées and dinner gatherings to add some courses that are useful and profitable, with a sauce of joyous and entertaining opinions, such that during the banquet one might even imagine the cruel spectacle of gladiators whose blood and guts ruined the clothing, stained the napkins, infected the food, and filled the glasses? Does not the Poet say:

---

[2] Guillaume Bouchet, *Les Serées*, ed. C.E. Roybet (Paris, 1873), vol. 4, p. 33. All translations are my own.

He who weds profit and pleasure
Artfully mixing the two in his writing
Instructing and pleasing the reader's mind
Wins the grand prize on all points, it seems to me.][3]

Les Serées can be said to have met these requirements with great fervor. Like the *Distaff Gospels*, *The Fifteen Joys of Marriage* that precedes and the *Caquets* that were to follow Bouchet's text (see Chapter 1), *Les Serées* indulges a large society of what I have led us to think of as proto-*salonniers* in folk wisdom, gossip, and hyperbole along with invocations of the most popular and respected experts in their topics of discussion. The sharing on the vagaries of the birthing body in particular are a delightful and vertiginous mix: from practical remedies for getting the postpartum body back in shape (for the continued pleasure of husbands), for example; to debates on how many months is optimal to carry a child to term; to the determining the sex of the child; to the effect of sight and imagination on fetal development; to fantastic tales of women who are rumored to have given birth without waking from a sound sleep! Popular fantasy runs cheek by jowl with the wisdom of the ancients and the moderns, incorporating multiple references to the likes of medical men such as Aristotle, Hippocrates, and Galen alongside the contemporaneous surgeons and obstetricians Paré and Joubert, the witch-hunters Spranger and Bodin, and the literary stratosphere from Sappho to Ronsard.

Bouchet pauses to remind us of the Aristotelian mandate of pleasing and instructing, interestingly, in the context of the birthing body, and he does so with dramatic comparison. So intriguing and potentially violent is the topic of the birthing and postpartum body, it seems, that the author likens the effect of its potential drama to that of a gladiatorial massacre, cups overrunning with blood, clothes stained with what appear to be bodily explosion—a most Rabelaisian entreaty into the corporeal indulgence of the violently regenerative body in the service of entertainment and even pleasure. Bouchet suggests by this comparison the poignancy and power of the realm of the body in reproduction and the host of dramatic and scrutinized outcomes to which it bears witness.

This presumption of the drama of the birthing body indeed motivated my study, impressed as I was with the range of instructive and pleasing narratives that its various scenarios across the early modern period embraces, and my progress through the stories has been not unlike Bouchet's. For its primary sources of authority and information, *Birthing Bodies* has mined the ancient texts of authors as far removed as Strabo, Hyginus, and Aristotle and paired them with both early modern literary luminaries from the Pléiade to the erudition of Madeleine and Catherine des Roches's mother–daughter poetic enterprise. To their voices was added the medical wisdom of the midwife Louise Boursier and several of the surgeons and obstetricians such as Ambroise Paré and Jacques Guillemeau with whom she both collaborated and collided. The voices of men and of women have

3 Bouchet, *Les Serées*, vol. 3, pp. 277–8.

been brought into this conversation, making of my text its own virtual salon of authors and readers, activists and political actors—the conventionally viable and normative alongside the inscrutable and condemned. With what I hope has been a responsible regard for both literary and historical context, I have suggested the ways in which understanding the birthing body of the early modern era might better inform some of the startlingly similar repermutations of the same issues of sex, gender, anxiety, and control that persist to this day.

What struck me most stunningly about Bouchet's lead-in to the "entertainment portion" of his *oeuvre*, as he might put it, was the very self-conscious declaration of literary pursuit: "Car tout ce qui se presentoit à nos yeux, ou qu'on entendoit dire, nous servoit de matiere & de livre" [Therefore all that was presented to our eyes and all that we heard tell, provided us with material for our book]. I share in the collective "nous servoit" of this sentiment. The gathering of texts and authors that are assembled in *Birthing Bodies* served me well in many of the same ways, both pleasing and instructive, it is hoped. Catherine des Roches's retelling of the dramatic tale of Agnodice, transvested and transported off to medical school to return and save her ailing sisters, was paired with the situation of both Catherine and her mother Madeleine who, by means of the powerful metaphor of the birthing body, reclaim a health for learned women, their literary progeny validated, promoted, and protected (Chapter 3, "Touching and Telling"); Louise Boursier served as a modern-day Agnodice, realizing and validating the gynecological wisdom proper to women, and mirroring the mother–daughter legacy: her *Instruction à ma fille* mirrors nicely the prefatorial refrain of the des Roches—"A ma fille," "A ma mère." Such reclaiming of women's agency in reproduction was also the intent of my pairing of Boursier with Rabelais (Chapter 2, "Staging the Competent Midwife"), wherein the fantastical stories of Gargantua (whose creator had ample knowledge of the medical wisdom and controversies of his day regarding the midwives he satirizes) are put in their place, as it were, by a royal midwife with, nonetheless, a robust sense of humor of her own. To this project of naming and reclaiming of the birthing body by women I added discussion of the appropriation of its generative and nutritive capacities by men (Chapter 1, "Spying at the Lying In," and Chapter 4, "Assimilation with a Vengeance"). Men as birthers, afterbirthers, breastfeeders—such are the improbable though surprisingly common rhetorical devices that the power of the reproductive corpus invoke, and with it a transgression of gender that appears to flount social norms while also reifying an unmistakably masculine hegemony. Finally, in ways that Bouchet might have found infinitely titillating and instructive, *Birthing Bodies* investigated the realms of corporeal inscrutability through parodies of the hermaphrodite (Chapter 5, "Unstable Bodies") and confounding accounts of birthing turned on its head from the New World (Chapter 6, "Strange Fellows in Bed").

It is hoped that this book has expanded the discussion of the early modern birthing "corpus" (in all its senses) so as to multiply rather than reduce its opportunities for apprehension and consideration. A book that dwells so heavily on men's narratives and male appropriation certainly runs the risk of overly determining the questions in ways that forestall a truly feminist critique of gender in this period. The opposite was surely my intent, though the recently deceased Mary Daly might certainly have called into question such an effort. Having invoked her as a foremother of my critical consciousness, I am reminded of the extent to which the gynocritical, gynocentric, indeed, gyno-exclusive mission was central to her re-envisioning and re-imagining of the world. Such, obviously, could not be my book.[4] My virtual "salon," as it were, would be, in the historical sense of the term, broader and would engage a range of genders and voices. There can be, of course, a nefariousness to appropriations of women's reproductive capacities (an injuriousness implied in the vengeance of assimilation evoked in Chapter 4); but I am also encouraged by more felicitous and capacious examples with regard to gender that question rather than re-entrench our view to misogyny of the past: Louise Boursier defending her rights as a medical professional; Jacques Duval defending the rights and lives of people born in indeterminate bodies; Catherine des Roches refusing wedlock and negotiating a (re)productive life in letters; and various reported examples, both pictorial (Magdalena Ventura, "the bearded mother"; the "bisexual" portrait of Francis I) and written, as in the couvade narratives from early modern explorers, which testify to a variety of lives in more generously gendered universes and serve to mitigate the undeniably heterosexist, heteronormative ideologies that held sway.

Were this book to seek an afterlife that attempted to theorize more deeply the impulses that govern men's appropriation of the birthing body, the couvade (as my investigation of even recent literature in Chapter 6 might suggest) would be its commencement. Aucassin's violent confrontation with the postpartum King of Torelore has always suggested two readings to me, one of self-loathing (Aucassin hating what he sees of himself in others) and one of envy: here is a view to a more permissive masculine life than he has been allowed—and therefore allowed himself—to indulge. Delving deeper into parturition envy and the embracing (instead of erasing) of women's experience is a gynecology for a more expansive, healthy, and liberated future.

***

The narrator of *Les Caquets de l'accouchée* set about his bedside mission in an effort to recover "sa pristine santé" [his original good health]. Being in the company of new mothers was purported to be a salutary pastime—restorative, instructive and, in no small way, entertaining. If *Birthing Bodies* has succeeded in any small way in better understanding our present by viewing the past, I would suggest one final contemporary example that may gain new meaning when viewed in the context of

[4] Mary Daly's obituary stresses the continuous stands she took (and the prices she paid) for insisting on teaching in exclusively female settings, even within coeducational institutions. See "Mary Daly, A Leader in Feminist Theology, Dies at 81," *The New York Times*, 7 January 2010, p. B18.

this study. David Carr's 2008 memoir of recovery from a desperate melancholy of his own relays this in homage to the maternal:

> Two years of reporting and a lot of awkward conversations later, I realized that in reductive psychoanalytic terms, I had achieved a measure of integration, not just between That Guy and This Guy but between my past and my present. Carl Jung suggested that until we embrace both our masculine and feminine sides, we can't be made whole. For all the testosterone I have deployed in my affairs, I experienced salvation in expressing common maternal behavior. You are always told to recover for yourself, but reproduction has an enormously simplifying effect on life: Are you willing to destroy others, including little babies, in order to feed the monster within?[5]

Guillaume Bouchet's more playful, though perhaps no less poignant evocation of the violence of certain narratives (all the more telling for being penned in the midst of the wars of religion), staged as it is in the context of women and their pregnant, birthing, and nurturing bodies, may well serve the likes of Carr and his readership in the attempt to link "past and present," "masculine and feminine" in more lasting, generous, and empowering ways. Such, at least, is the legacy that a book such as this has attempted to generate.

[5] David Carr, "Me and My Girls," *The New York Times Magazine*, 20 July 2008, p. 54.

Bibliography

Texts before 1800

Artus, Thomas. *L'Isle des hermaphrodites* [1605]. Ed. Claude-Gilbert Dubois. Geneva: Droz, 1996.

Aubigné, Théodore Agrippa de. *Les Tragiques* [1616]. Ed. A. Garnier and J. Plattard. Paris: Société des Textes Français Modernes, 1990.

Aucassin et Nicolette. Ed. Mario Roques. Paris: Champion, 1982.

Biet, Antoine. *Voyage de la France équinoxiale en lisle de Cayenne, entrepris par les François en l'année* MDCLII–1664. Paris: F. Clouzier, 1664.

Boaistuau, Pierre. *Histoires prodigieuses les plus mémorables qui ayent esté observées depuis la nativité de Jésus-Christ, jusques à nostre siècle: extraictes de plusieurs fameux autheurs grecz et latins, sacrez et prophanes*. Paris: Vincent Sertenas, 1560.

——, Claude Tesserant, and François de Belleforest. *Histoires prodigieuses les plus mémorable qui ayent esté observées depuis la nativité de Jésus-Christ, jusques à nostre siècle: extraictes de plusieurs fameux autheurs grecz et latins, sacrez et prophanes*. Paris: Veuve de Gabriel Buon, 1598.

Bouchet, Guillaume. *Les Serées* [1584-98]. Ed. C.E. Roybet. Paris: Alphonse Lemerre, 1873.

Boursier, Louise (Bourgeois). *Observations diverses, sur la sterilité, perte de fruits, foecondité, accouchements, et maladies des femmes et enfants nouveaux-nés* [1609]. Ed. Françoise Olive. Paris: Côté-femmes, 1992.

——. *Observations diverses, sur la sterilité, perte de fruict, foecondité, accouchements, et maladies des femmes et enfants nouveaux naiz*. Paris: Melchior Mondière, 1626.

——. *Récit véritable de la naissance de messeigneurs et dames les enfans de France; Instruction à ma fille et autres textes*. Ed. François Rouget and Colette Winn. Geneva: Droz, 2000.

Les Caquets de l'accouchée: recueil général suivi de l'Anti-Caquet, des Essais de Mathurine et de la Sentence par corps. Paris: C. Marpon and E. Flammarion, 1890.

Les Caquets de l'accouchée [1622]. Ed. Edouard Fournier. Introduction, M. Le Roux de Lincy. Paris: P. Jannet, 1855.

C'est la deduction du sumptueux ordre, plaisantz spectacles et magnifiques theatres dresses, et exhibes par les citoiens de Rouen... Rouen, 1551.

Des Roches, Madeleine Neveu, and Catherine Fredonnoit. *Les Oeuvres* [1579]. Ed. Anne R. Larsen. Geneva: Droz, 1993.

——. *Les Secondes oeuvres* [1583]. Ed. Anne R. Larsen. Geneva: Droz, 1998.

——. *Les Missives* [1586]. Ed. Anne R. Larsen. Geneva: Droz, 1999.

——. *From Mother and Daughter: poems, dialogues, and letters of les dames des Roches/Madeleine and Catherine des Roches*. Ed. and trans. Anne R. Larsen. Chicago: University of Chicago Press, 2006.

The Distaff Gospels: A First Modern English Edition of Les Evangiles des quenouilles [includes the original French]. Ed. and trans. Madeleine Jeay and Kathleen Garay. Peterborough, Ontario: Broadview Press, 2006.

Du Bellay, Joachim. *La Deffence et illustration de la langue Françoyse*. Ed. H. Chamard, Paris: Société des Textes Français Modernes, 1970.

——. *Les Regrets*. Ed. Françoise Joukovsky. Paris: Garnier Flammarion, 1971.

——. *Les Regrets*. Trans. C.H. Sisson. Manchester: Carcanet Press, 1984.

Du Tertre, Jean-Baptiste. *Histoire générale des isles de S. Christophe, de la Guadeloupe, de la Martinique et autres dans l'Amérique*. Paris: J. Langlois, 1654.

Duval, Jacques. *Des Hermaphrodits, accouchemens des femmes et traitement qui est requis pour les relever en santé, et bien élever leurs enfans*. Rouen: David Geuffroy, 1612.

L'Entrée de Henri II à Rouen 1550. Ed. Margaret M. McGowan. Amsterdam: Theatrum Orbis Terrarum, 1974.

Erasmus, Desiderius. *Collected Works of Erasmus*. Ed. J.K. Sowards. Toronto: University of Toronto Press, 1985.

Foigny, Gabriel de. *The Southern Land Known* [*La Terre Australe Connue*, 1676]. Ed. and trans. David Fausett. Syracuse, NY: Syracuse University Press, 1993.

Garasse, François. *La Doctrine curieuse des beaux esprits de ce temps ou prétendus tels*. Paris: S. Chappelet, 1624.

Guillemeau, Jacques. *De l'Heureux accouchement des femmes où il est traicté du gouvernement de leur grossesse, de leur travail naturel et contre nature, du traictement estant accouchées et de leurs maladies*. Paris: Nicolas Buon, 1609.

——. *Child-birth or, The Happy Deliverie of Women*. Anonymous translation. London: A. Hatfield, 1612. Reprint: Amsterdam: Theatrum Orbins Terrarum, 1972.

Hecquet, Philippe. *De l'Indécence aux hommes d'accoucher les femmes et de l'obligation aux mères de nourrir leurs enfants* [1707]. Paris: Côté-femmes, 1990.

Hyginus, Gaius Julius. *Fabulae*. Ed. Peter K. Marshall. Munich: Walter de Gruyter, 2002.

——. *Fables*. Ed. and trans. Jean-Yves Boriaud. Paris: Les Belles lettres, 1997.

——. *The Myths of Hyginus*. Ed. and trans. Mary Grant. Lawrence: University of Kansas Press, 1960.

Joubert, Laurent. *La Médecine et le régime de santé: des erreurs populaires et propos vulgaires* [1578–79]. 2 vols. Ed. Madeleine Tiollais. Paris: L'Harmattan, 1997.

Kramer, Heinrich, and James Sprenger. *The Malleus Maleficarum* [c. 1490]. Ed. and trans. Montague Summers. New York: Dover, 1971.

La Touche, Gervais de. *La Tres-haute et Tres-souveraine science de l'art et industrie naturelle d'enfanster. Contre La Maudicte et Perverse Impericie des femmes que l'on appelle saiges femmes, ou belles meres, lesquelles par leur ignorance font journellement perir une infinité de femmes d'enfans à l'enfantement*. Paris: Didier Millot, 1587.

Mauquest de La Motte, Guillaume. *Traité complet des accouchemens naturels, non naturels et contre nature, expliqué dans un grand nombre d'observations et de réflexions sur l'art d'accoucher* ... Paris: L. d'Houry, 1721.

Montaigne, Michel de. *Oeuvres complètes*. Ed. Albert Thibaudet and Maurice Rat. Paris: Gallimard, 1962.

——. *Essais*, livre 2. Ed. Alexandre Micha. Paris: Garnier-Flammarion, 1969.

——. *The Complete Works of Montaigne*. Trans. Donald M. Frame. Stanford: Stanford University Press, 1976.

——. *Essais*. Ed. Pierre Villey. Paris: Presses Universitaires de France, 1978.

Ovid. *The Metamorphoses*, Book III. Trans. Frank Justus Miller. Cambridge, MA: Harvard University Press, 1916 [reprinted 1984].

Paré, Ambroise. *Deux livres de chirurgie, de la génération de l'homme, & manière d'extraire les enfans hors du ventre de la mère, ensemble ce qu'il faut faire pour la faire mieux, & plus tost accoucher, avec la cure de plusieurs maladies qui luy peuvent survenir*. Paris: André Wechel, 1573.

——. *Les Oeuvres d'Ambroise Paré* ... 9th edn. Lyon: Vve de C. Rigaud et C. Obert, 1633.

——. *Des Monstres et prodiges*. Ed. Jean Céard. Geneva: Droz, 1971.

Pizan, Christine de. *Le Livre de la cité des dames*. Ed. and trans. Eric Hicks and Thérèse Moreau. Paris: Stock, 1986.

Les Quinze joies de mariage. Ed. and trans. Monique Santucci. Paris: Stock, 1986.

Rabelais, François. *The Complete Works of François Rabelais*. Trans. Donald M. Frame. Berkeley: University of California Press, 1991.

——. *Oeuvres complètes*. Ed. Mireille Huchon. Paris: Gallimard, 1994.

Ronsard, Pierre de. *Oeuvres complètes*. Ed. Jean Céard, Daniel Ménager, and Michel Simonin. Paris: Gallimard, 1993.

Scève, Maurice. *Délie* [1544]. Ed. Françoise Charpentier. Paris: Gallimard, 1984.

Schmidt, Albert-Marie, ed. *Poètes du XVIe siècle*. Paris: Gallimard, 1953.

Sébillet, Thomas. *Art Poétique* [1548]. Ed. F. Gaiffe and F. Goyet. Paris: Nizet, 1988.

La Seconde après-dînée du caquet de l'accouchée et autres facéties du temps de Louis XIII [1622]. Ed. Alain Mercier. Paris: Honoré Champion, 2003.

Strabo. *Geographia*, Book III. Trans. H.L. Jones. Cambridge, MA: Harvard University Press, 1969.

Thevet, André. *Le Brésil d'André Thevet: Les Singularités de la France Antarctique* [1557]. Ed. Frank Lestringant. Paris: Editions Chandeigne, 1997.
——. *Singularitez de la France antarctique*. Paris: Chez les héritiers de Maurice de La Porte, 1558.
——. *La Cosmographie universelle*. 2 vols. Paris: Ct. Chaudière, 1575.
Vives, Juan Luis. *A very fruteful and pleasant boke callyd the instruction of a Christen woman*. Trans. Richard Hyrde. London: Thomas Berth, 1541.
——. *Livre de l'institution de la Femme Chriestienne*. Trans. Pierre de Changy. Le Havre: Lemale et Compagnie, 1891. Reprint: Geneva: Slatkine, 1970.
——. *The Education of a Christian Woman: A Sixteenth-Century Manual*. Ed. and trans. Charles Fantazzi. Chicago: University of Chicago Press, 2000.

Secondary Sources

Abel, Elizabeth, ed. *Writing and Sexual Difference*. Chicago: University of Chicago Press, 1982.
Andreae, Bernard. *The Art of Rome*. Trans. Robert Erich Wolf. New York: Harry N. Abrams, 1977.
Antonioli, Roland. *Rabelais et la médecine*. Geneva: Droz, 1976.
Bakhtin, Mikhail. *Rabelais and His World*. Trans. Hélène Iswolsky. Bloomington: Indiana University Press, 1984.
Baraz, Michaël. *Rabelais et la joie de la liberté*. Paris: Corti, 1983.
Beasley, Faith E. *Revising Memory: Women's Fiction and Memoirs in Seventeenth-Century France*. New Brunswick, NJ: Rutgers University Press, 1990.
——. *Salons, History, and the Creation of Seventeenth-Century France: Mastering Memory*. Aldershot: Ashgate, 2006.
Beauvoir, Simone de. *Le Deuxième sexe*. Paris: Gallimard, 1949.
——. *The Second Sex*. Trans. H.M. Parshley. New York: Vintage, 1974.
Berriot-Salvadore, Evelyne. *Les Femmes dans la société française de la Renaissance*. Geneva: Droz, 1990.
——. *Un Corps, un Destin: La femme dans la médecine de la Renaissance*. Paris: Honoré Champion, 1993.
Berry, Philippa. *Of Chastity and Power: Elizabethan Literature and the Unmarried Queen*. London: Routledge, 1989.
Bhabha, Homi. "Are You a Man or a Mouse?" in *Constructing Masculinity*. Ed. Maurice Berger, Brian Wallis, and Simon Watson, pp. 57–65. New York: Routledge, 1995.
Bicks, Caroline. "Midwiving Virility in Early Modern England," in *Maternal Measures: Figuring Caregiving in the Early Modern Period*. Ed. Naomi J. Miller and Naomi Yavneh, pp. 49–64. Aldershot: Ashgate, 2000.
——. *Midwiving Subjects in Shakespeare's England*. Aldershot: Ashgate, 2003.

Blumenfeld-Kosinski, Renate. *Not of Woman Born: Representations of Caesarean Birth in Medieval and Renaissance Culture*. Ithaca, NY: Cornell University Press, 1990.

Bordo, Susan. "The Body and the Reproduction of Femininity," in *Writing on the Body: Female Embodiment and Feminist Theory*. Ed. Katie Conboy, Nadia Medina, and Sarah Stanbury, pp. 90–110. New York: Columbia University Press, 1997.

Breitenberg, Mark. *Anxious Masculinity in Early Modern England*. Cambridge: Cambridge University Press, 1996.

Brennan, Arthur, Susan Ayers, Hafez Ahmed, and Sylvie Marshall-Lucette. "A Critical Review of the Couvade Syndrome: The Pregnant Male." *Journal of Reproductive and Infant Psychology*, 25/3 (2007): 173–89.

Broomhall, Susan. *Women's Medical Work in Early Modern France*. Manchester: Manchester University Press, 2004.

Bronski, Michael. *The Pleasure Principle: Sex, Backlash, and the Struggle for Gay Freedom*. New York: St Martin's Press, 1998.

Butler, Judith. *Undoing Gender*. New York: Routledge, 2004.

Bynum, Caroline Walker. *Jesus as Mother: Studies in the Spirituality of the High Middle Ages*. Berkeley: University of California Press, 1984.

——. *Fragmentation and Redemption: Essays on Gender and the Human Body in Medieval Religion*. New York: Zone Books, 1992.

Cady, Joseph. "The 'Masculine Love' of the 'Princes of Sodom' 'Practising the Art of Ganymede' at Henri III's Court: The Homosexuality of Henri III and His Mignons in Pierre de L'Estoiles' *Mémoires-Journaux*," in *Desire and Discipline: Sex and Sexuality in the Premodern West*. Ed. Jacqueline Murray and Konrad Eisenbichler, pp. 123–54. Toronto: University of Toronto Press, 1996.

Carr, David. "Me and My Girls." *The New York Times Magazine*. 20 July 2008: p. 54.

Céard, Jean. *La Nature et les prodiges*. Geneva: Droz, 1977.

Certeau, Michel de. *The Writing of History*. New York: Columbia University Press, 1988.

Chase, Cheryl. "Hermaphrodites with Attitude: Mapping the Emergence of Intersex Political Activism." *Journal of Lesbian and Gay Studies*, 4/2 (1998): 189–211.

Conboy, Katie, Nadia Medina, and Sarah Stanbury, eds. *Writing on the Body: Female Embodiment and Feminist Theory*. New York: Columbia University Press, 1997.

Crawford, Katherine B. "Love, Sodomy, and Scandal: Controlling the Sexual Reputation of Henry III." *Journal of the History of Sexuality*, 12 (2003): 513–42.

Daly, Mary. *Gyn/Ecology: The Metaethics of Radical Feminism*. Boston, MA: Beacon Press, 1978.

Daston, Lorraine, and Katharine Park. "The Hermaphrodite and the Orders of Nature: Sexual Ambiguity in Early Modern France." *Gay and Lesbian Quarterly*, 1 (1995): 419–38.

Dawson, Warren R. *The Custom of the Couvade*. Manchester: Manchester University Press, 1929. Reprinted in Nor Hall and Warren R. Dawson. *Broodmales: A Psychological Essay on Men in Childbirth*. Dallas: Spring Publications, 1989.

DeJean, Joan. *Tender Geographies: Women and the Origins of the Novel in France*. New York: Columbia University Press, 1991.

Diller, Georges E. *Les Dames des Roches: Etude sur la vie littéraire à Poitiers dans la deuxième moitié du XVIème siècle*. Paris: Droz, 1936.

Dobbie, B.M. Wilmott. "An Attempt to Estimate the True Rate of Maternal Mortality, Sixteenth to Eighteenth Centuries." *Medical History*, 26 (1982): 79–90.

Duval, Edwin M. *The Design of Rabelais's* Pantagruel. New Haven, CT: Yale University Press, 1991.

Ezell, Margaret. *Writing Women's Literary History*. Baltimore, MD: The Johns Hopkins University Press, 1993.

Ferguson, Gary. *Queer (Re)Readings in the French Renaissance: Homosexuality, Gender, Culture*. Aldershot: Ashgate, 2008.

Ferguson, Margaret W., Maureen Quilligan, and Nancy Vickers, eds. *Rewriting the Renaissance: The Discourses of Sexual Difference in Early Modern Europe*. Chicago: University of Chicago Press, 1986.

Finucci, Valeria, and Kevin Brownlee, eds. *Generation and Degeneration: Tropes of Reproduction in Literature and History from Antiquity to Early Modern Europe*. Durham, NC: Duke University Press, 2001.

Fisher, Will. "The Renaissance Beard: Masculinity in Early Modern England." *Renaissance Quarterly*, 54/1 (Spring 2001): 155–87.

Freud, Sigmund. *The Freud Reader*, Ed. Peter Gay. New York: Norton, 1989.

Friedman, Susan Stanford. "Creativity and the Childbirth Metaphor: Gender Difference in Literary Discourse." *Feminist Studies*, 13/1 (1987): 49–82.

Gélis, Jacques. *History of Childbirth* [*L'Arbre et le fruit*, 1984]. Trans. Rosemary Morris. Boston, MA: Northeastern University Press, 1991.

Gillet, Louis. "Jusepe de Ribera." *The Catholic Encyclopedia*. 13. New York: Robert Appleton Company, 1912. 12 May 2008. http://www.newadvent.org/cathen/13031b.htm.

Glidden, Hope. *The Storyteller as Humanist:* The Serées *of Guillaume Bouchet*. Lexington, KY: French Forum, 1981.

Gubar, Susan. "'The Blank Page' and the Issues of Female Creativity," in *Writing and Sexual Difference*. Ed. Elizabeth Abel, pp. 73–93. Chicago: University of Chicago Press, 1982.

——. *Judas: A Biography*. New York: W.W. Norton, 2009.

Hampton, Cathy. "Unpicking Female Exemplarity; or, The Usefulness of Body Stories: Reassessing Female Communal Identity in Two Early Modern French Texts." *Modern Language Review*, 102 (2007): 381–96.

Jacobus, Mary. "Incorruptible Milk: Breast-feeding and the French Revolution," in *Rebel Daughters: Women and the French Revolution*. Ed. S. Melzer and L. Rabine, pp. 54–75. Oxford: Oxford University Press, 1992.

Jacques, Jean-Marie. "Sur l'accouchement de Gargamelle." *Bulletin de l'Association des amis de Rabelais et de La Devinière*, 4/10 (1991): 396–400.

Janier, André. *Les "Serées," 1584, 1597, 1598, du librairie-imprimeur Guillaume Bouchet (1514–1594)*. Paris: Honoré Champion, 2006.

Jones, Ann Rosalind. "Assimilation with a Difference: Renaissance Women Poets and Literary Influence." *Yale French Studies*, 62 (1981): 135–53.

——. *The Currency of Eros: Women's Love Lyric in Europe, 1540–1620*. Bloomington: Indiana University Press, 1990.

Jordan, Constance. *Renaissance Feminism: Literary Texts and Political Models*. Ithaca, NY: Cornell University Press, 1990.

Jordan, Mark D. *The Invention of Sodomy in Christian Theology*. Chicago: University of Chicago Press, 1997.

Jusepe de Ribera: lo Spagnoletto 1591–1652. Fort Worth, TX: Kimball Art Museum, 1982.

Kessler, Suzanne J. "The Medical Construction of Gender: Case Management of Intersexed Infants." *Signs: Journal of Women in Culture and Society*, 16 (1990): 3–26.

King, Helen. "Agnodike and the Profession of Medicine." *Proceedings of the Cambridge Philological Society*, 32 (1986): 53–77.

King, Margaret. *Women of the Renaissance*. Chicago: University of Chicago Press, 1991.

Klein, Hilary. "Couvade Syndrome: Male Counterpart to Pregnancy." *International Journal of Psychiatry in Medicine*, 21/1 (1991): 57–69.

Klein, Joan Larsen, ed. *Daughters, Wives and Widows: Writings by Men about Women and Marriage*. Chicago: University of Illinois Press, 1992.

Labalme, Patricia H., ed. *Beyond Their Sex: Learned Women of the European* Past. New York: New York University Press, 1984.

LaGuardia, David P. *Intertextual Masculinity in French Renaissance Literature: Rabelais, Brantôme, and the* Cent nouvelles nouvelles. Aldershot: Ashgate, 2008.

Laqueur, Thomas. *Making Sex: The Body and Gender from the Greeks to Freud*. Cambridge, MA: Harvard University Press, 1990.

Larsen, Anne R., and Colette Winn. *Renaissance Women Writers: French Texts/American Contexts*. Detroit, MI: Wayne State University, 1994.

Larsen, Anne R. "Catherine des Roches' 'Epistre A Sa Mere' (1579)." *Allegorica*, 7/2 (1984): 58–64.

——. "Reading/Writing Gender in the Renaissance: The Case of Catherine des Roches (1542–1587)." *Symposium*, 41/4 (1987–88): 292–307.

Lestringant, Frank. *Mapping the Renaissance World: The Geographical Imagination in the Age of Discovery*. Trans. David Fausett. Berkeley: University of California Press, 1994.

——. *Cannibals: The Discovery and Representation of the Cannibal from Columbus to Jules Verne* [*Le Cannibale: grandeur et décadence*, 1994]. Trans. Rosemary Morris. Berkeley: University of California Press, 1997.

Long, Kathleen P. ed. "Motherhood and Martyrdom in the Poetry of Théodore Agrippa d'Aubigné." *Neophilologus*, 76/2 (1992): 198–211.

——. *High Anxiety: Masculinity in Crisis in Early Modern* France. Kirksville, MO: Truman State University Press, 2002.

——. *Hermaphrodites in Renaissance Europe*. Aldershot: Ashgate, 2006.

—— ed. *Gender and Scientific Discourse in Early Modern Culture*. Aldershot: Ashgate, 2010.

Longman, Jeré. "South African Runner's Sex-Verification Result Won't Be Public." *The New York Times*. 19 November 2009.

Luborsky, Ruth. "The Pictoral Image of the Jew in Elizabethan Secular Books." *Shakespeare Quarterly*, 46/4 (Winter 1995): 449–53.

Marshall, Sherrin, ed. *Women in Reformation and Counter-Reformation Europe: Public and Private Worlds*. Bloomington: Indiana University Press, 1989.

Matthews Grieco, Sara F. *Ange ou Diablesse: La représentation de la femme au XVIe siècle*. Paris: Flammarion, 1991.

Maus, Katharine Eisaman. "A Womb of His Own: Male Renaissance Poets in the Female Body," in *Sexuality and Gender in Early Modern Europe: Institutions, Texts, Images*. Ed. James Grantham Turner, pp. 266–88. Cambridge: Cambridge University Press, 1993.

McCoskey, Denise Eileen. "Gender at the Crossroads of Empire: Locating Women in Strabo's *Geography*," in *Strabo's Cultural Geography: The Making of a Kolossourgia*. Ed. Daniela Dueck, Hugh Lindsay, and Sarah Pothecary, pp. 56–72. Cambridge: Cambridge University Press, 2005.

McTavish, Lianne. *Childbirth and the Display of Authority in Early Modern France*. Aldershot: Ashgate, 2005.

Meyer, Barbara Hochstetler. "Marguerite de Navarre and the Androgynous Portrait of François Ier." *Renaissance Quarterly*, 48/2 (1995): 287–325.

Miller, Naomi J., and Naomi Yavneh, eds. *Maternal Measures: Figuring Caregiving in the Early Modern Period*. Aldershot: Ashgate, 2000.

Montrose, Louis. "The Work of Gender in the Discourse of Discovery," in *New World Encounters*. Ed. Stephen Greenblatt, pp. 177–217. Berkeley: University of California Press, 1993.

Morgan, Jennifer. *Laboring Women: Reproduction and Gender in New World Slavery*. Philadelphia: University of Pennsylvania Press, 2004.

Park, Katharine, and Robert A. Nye. "Destiny is Anatomy." *The New Republic*, 18 (February 1991): 53–7.

Parker, Patricia. "Gender Ideology, Gender Change: The Case of Marie Germain." *Critical Inquiry*, 19/2 (1993): 337–64.

Perkins, Wendy. *Midwifery and Medicine in Early Modern France: Louise Bourgeois*. Exeter: Exeter University Press, 1996.

Perkinson, Jim. "The Body of White Space: Beyond Stiff Voices, Flaccid Feelings, and Silent Cells," in *Revealing Male Bodies*. Ed. Nancy Tuana, William Cowling, Maurice Hamington, Greg Johnson, and Terrance MacMullan, pp. 173–97. Bloomington: Indiana University Press, 2002.

Perry, Ruth. "Colonizing the Breast: Sexuality and Maternity in Eighteenth-Century England," in *Forbidden History: The State, Society, and the Regulation of Sexuality in Modern Europe*. Ed. John C. Fout, pp. 107–37. Chicago: University of Chicago Press, 1992.

Pomata, Gianna. "Menstruating Men: Similarity and Difference of the Sexes in Early Modern Medicine," in *Generation and Degeneration: Tropes of Reproduction in Literature and History from Antiquity to Early Modern Europe*. Ed. Valeria Finucci and Kevin Brownlee, pp. 109–52. Durham, NC: Duke University Press, 2001.

Read, Kirk. "Mother's Milk from Father's Breast: Maternity without Women in Male French Renaissance Lyric," in *High Anxiety: Masculinity in Crisis in Early Modern France*. Ed. Kathleen P. Long, pp. 71–92. Kirksville, MO: Truman State University Press, 2002.

——. "Staging the Competent Midwife: Louise Boursier as Response to François Rabelais's Gargantuan Birth," in *Esprit généreux, esprit pantagruélicque: Essays by His Students in Honor of François Rigolot*. Ed. Leushuis, Reinier, and Zahi Zalloua, pp. 141–58. Geneva: Droz, 2008.

Reeser, Todd. *Moderating Masculinity in Early Modern Culture*. Chapel Hill: University of North Carolina Press, 2006.

Rigolot, François. "Rabelais, Misogyny, and Christian Charity: Biblical Intertextuality and the Renaissance Crisis of Exemplarity." *PMLA*, 109/2 (1994): 225–37.

Rose, Mary Beth, ed. *Women in the Middle Ages and the Renaissance: Literary and Historical Perspectives*. Syracuse, NY: Syracuse University Press, 1986.

Sankovitch, Tilde. *French Women Writers and the Book: Myths of Access and Desire*. Syracuse, NY: Syracuse University Press, 1988.

Schiebinger, Londa. "Competing Cosmologies: Locating Sex and Gender in the Natural Order," in *The Mind Has No Sex? Women in the Origins of Modern Science*. Ed. Londa Schiebinger, pp. 160–88. Cambridge, MA: Harvard University Press, 1989.

——. *Nature's Body: Gender in the Making of Modern Science*. Boston, MA: Beacon Press, 1993.

Schofield, Roger. "Did the Mothers Really Die? Three Centuries of Maternal Mortality in 'The World We Have Lost'," in *The World We Have Gained: Histories of Population and Social Structure*. Ed. Lloyd Bonfield, Richard Smith, and Keith Wrightson, pp. 231–60. New York: Blackwell Publishers, 1986.

Sedgwick, Eve Kosofsky. *Between Men: English Literature and Male Homosocial Desire*. New York: Columbia University Press, 1985.

Showalter, Elaine. "Toward a Feminist Poetics," in *The New Feminist Criticism: Essays on Women, Literature and Theory*. Ed. Elaine Showalter, pp. 125–43. New York: Pantheon, 1985.

Stanton, Domna. "Recuperating Women and the Man behind the Screen," in *Sexuality and Gender in Early Modern Europe: Institutions, Texts, Images*. Ed. James Grantham Turner, pp. 247–65. Cambridge: Cambridge University Press, 1993.

Steinberg, Leo, *The Sexuality of Christ in Renaissance Art and in Modern Oblivion*. 2nd edn. Chicago: University of Chicago Press, 1996.

Stone, Lawrence. *The Family, Sex, and Marriage in England 1500–1800*. New York: Harper and Row, 1977.

Stone, Sandy. "The Empire Strikes Back: A Posttranssexual Manifesto," in *Writing on the Body: Female Embodiment of Feminist Theory*. Ed. Katie Conboy, Nadia Medina, and Sarah Stanbury, pp. 337–59. New York: Columbia University Press, 1997.

Timmermans, Linda. *L'Access des femmes à la culture (1598–1715)*. Paris: Champion, 1993.

Trebay, Guy. "He's Pregnant. You're Speechless." *The New York Times*. 22 June 2008.

Turner, James Grantham. ed. *Sexuality and Gender in Early Modern Europe: Institutions, Texts, Images*. Cambridge: Cambridge University Press, 1993.

——. *Schooling Sex: Libertine Literature and Erotic Education in Italy, France, and England 1534*–1685. London: Oxford University Press, 2003.

Velasco, Sherry. *Male Delivery: Reproduction, Effeminacy, and Pregnant Men in Early Modern Spain*. Nashville, TN: Vanderbilt University Press, 2006.

Virtue, Nancy E. "Translation as Violation: A Reading of Pierre Boaistuau's *Histoires tragiques*." *Renaissance and Reformation/Renaissance et Réforme*, 22/3 (1998): 35–7.

Waddington, Raymond B. "The Bisexual Portrait of Francis I: Fontainebleau, Castiglione, and the Tone of Courtly Mythology," in *Playing with Gender: A Renaissance Pursuit*. Ed. Jean Brink, Maryanne C. Horowitz, and Allison P. Coudert, pp. 99–132. Urbana: University of Illinois Press, 1991.

Watson, Foster. *Vives and the Renascence Education of Women*. New York: Longmans, 1912.

Whatley, Janet. "Savage Hierarchies: French Catholic Observers of the New World." *Sixteenth Century Journal*, 1/3 (1986): 319–30.

Wiesner, Merry E. *Women and Gender in Early Modern Europe*. Cambridge: Cambridge University Press, 1993.

Wintroub, Michael. *A Savage Mirror: Power, Identity, and Knowledge in Early Modern France*. Stanford, CA: Stanford University Press, 2006.

Worth-Stylianou, Valérie. *Les Traités d'obstétrique en langue française au seuil de la modernité*. Geneva: Droz, 2007.

Zapperi, Roberto. *The Pregnant Man*. Trans. Brian Williams. Chur, Switzerland: Harwood Academic Publishers, 1991.

Index